Let's Talk About PANS/PANDAS

A Guide for Parents and Kids

Dr. Kimberly Brayman
Licensed Psychologist #2464

& Dr. Isaac Melamed, MD
Immunologist

Illustrated by

Irina Denissova

ISBN (paperback) 978-1-951688-52-3

EPUB ISBN 978-1-951688-50-9

Foreword

Pediatric acute-onset neuropsychiatric syndrome (PANS) is a disease that dramatically affects children and their families. Because of its acute onset, many parents and caregivers find themselves with few tools to mitigate the effect of this disease on their children's lives.

In my practice, I have successfully treated hundreds of children from a clinical standpoint. I have also had the pleasure of working with Dr. Brayman in her work as a psychologist and neurofeedback professional.

In this book, she provides practical and effective strategies for parents and children as they work to maintain a healthy lifestyle with this challenging diagnosis.

This book is a "must read" for any family struggling with this challenging disease.

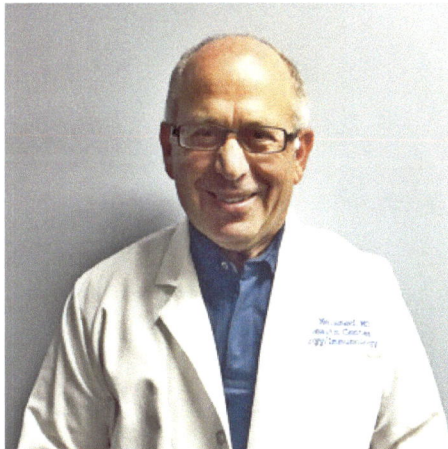

Isaac Melamed, MD

Dr. Isaac Melamed is currently a clinician in private practice in the metro Denver area of Colorado. Previously, he was in academia in the US, Canada and Israel. His focus is the interaction between the immune and nervous system – neuro-immune connection publishing over 150 papers, presenting and lecturing around the world.

He also founded an independent clinical research facility, IMMUNOe Research Center, and has been a principle investigator on over 250 clinical trials. His major areas of interest are cross-talk between the nervous and immune system, the role of the immune system in neuro-inflammatory diseases, and cytoskeletal signaling.

Dr. Melamed has presented and lectured in the United States and overseas. On account of his achievements, he received an Award of Clinical Immunology Society in 2002, Research Award of the American Academy of Allergy and Immunology in 1993, honorable certificate in 1991, and the Tisdale Award for Excellence in Research in 1990.

Introduction

Pediatric Acute-onset Neuropsychiatric Syndrome (PANS) is a clinically diverse disorder with several different causes and mechanisms.

Diagnosis is made based on the abrupt onset of obsessive-compulsive (OC) symptoms and/or restricted eating behaviors, with at least two of these symptoms:

- anxiety, emotional liability and/or depression
- irritability/ oppositionality/ aggression
- behavior regression
- deterioration in school performance
- sensory or motor abnormalities, and
- somatic symptoms.

Pediatric Autoimmune Neuropsychiatric Disorders (PANDAS) is a subset of PANS. It is specifically associated with streptococcal infections. Many of the symptoms are the same.

PANS and PANDAS are diagnoses of exclusion. This means a comprehensive diagnostic evaluation is needed, to rule out other neurological or psychiatric conditions.

Treatment for PANS/PANDAS should be individualized to your child's specific symptoms. Treatments involve

- targeting specific infection
- treating autoimmune and inflammatory issues (particularly brain inflammation), and
- working to prevent further relapses.

More than 80% of PANS patients have immune system abnormalities/ deficiencies. Treating these may be part of your child's treatment plan.

Psychiatric treatment (from a psychiatrist familiar with PANS/PANDAS) may be needed to address issues of anxiety, depression (including suicidality), out of control anger, obsessive-compulsive issues, and emotional lability.

A psychologist will support and treat the child, and the family. They will help with behavioral intervention, coping skills, teaching strategies, and processing everyone's feelings. Cognitive behavioral therapy is the treatment of choice for mood disorders. The use of technology-driven treatments such as neurofeedback and apps to track mood and behavior are increasingly useful.

Please ask your treatment team for more specific resources.

This book is written for your child, with a little wisdom in it for you. Take a breath, slowly let it out – let's talk about PANS/PANDAS.

Contents

My body is amazing...

You have an amazing body that helps you do really cool things!

Can you walk, run, and jump?

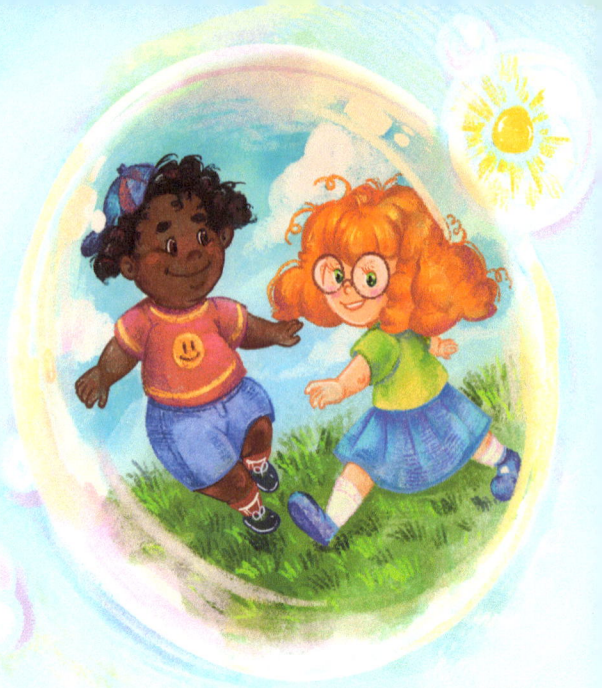

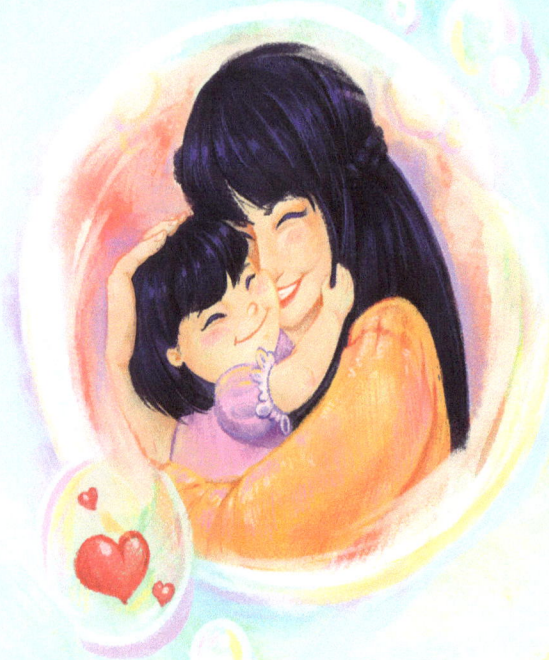

Can you hug your mom?

Do you ride a bicycle, kick a ball, climb the monkey bars?

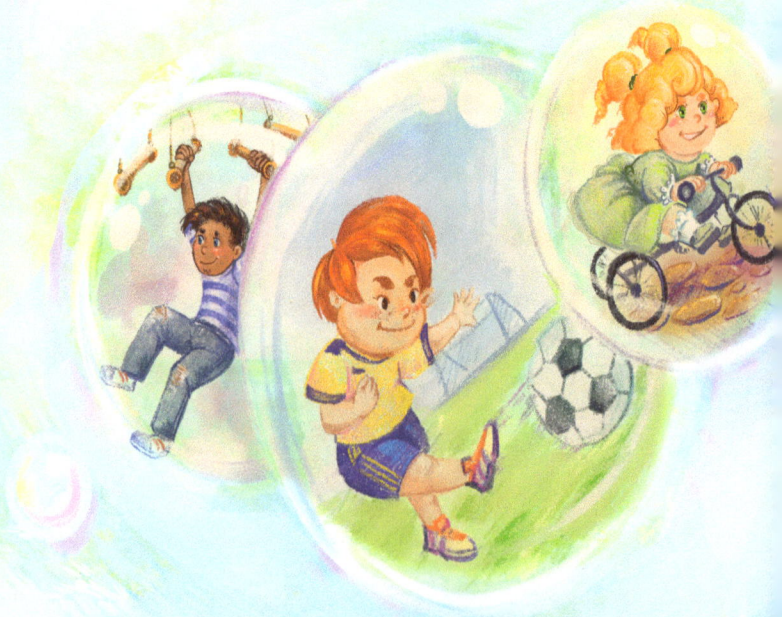

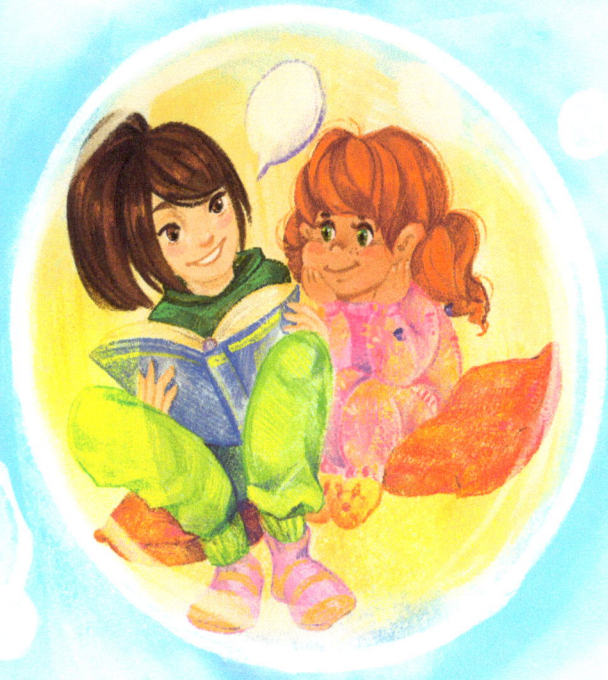

Do you listen to stories, or read them to yourself?

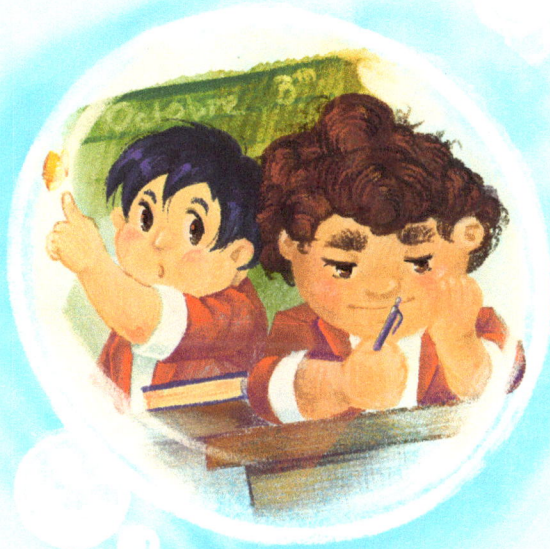

Do you go to school to learn, or learn at home?

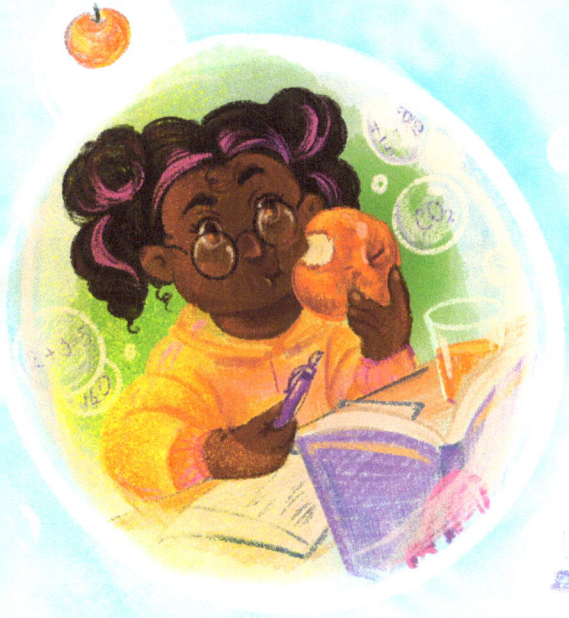

You are amazing! No one else is like you.

Oh, no! What is happening to me?

Sometimes, things go wrong in our bodies. How we feel and act changes very quickly.

Our brains are our control centers. Pathways connect brain to all the different parts of our body. Information goes back and forth, and our defenses get activated when they are needed.

You can suddenly just feel YUCKY! A virus, bacteria or other invader can make you sick.

Usually that means you have a runny nose, a cough, a fever, a rash, a headache or an upset tummy for a day or two. Your brain tells your immune system, "Fight the germs and get this body healthy again!"

Sometimes our brain gets mixed up, though, and all kinds of things go wrong.

Parents can help

A sick child feels out of control.

The more control (or choices) a child has, the less they try to control the things they can't.

How can you, as a parent, stay calm, positive, and give *many* more choices? Work on this.

Having huge emotions feels out of control! Your child is reacting to how *they* feel – and to how you handle things, even the tough stuff.

It helps when you respond consciously, instead of reacting emotionally.

Work on staying calm.

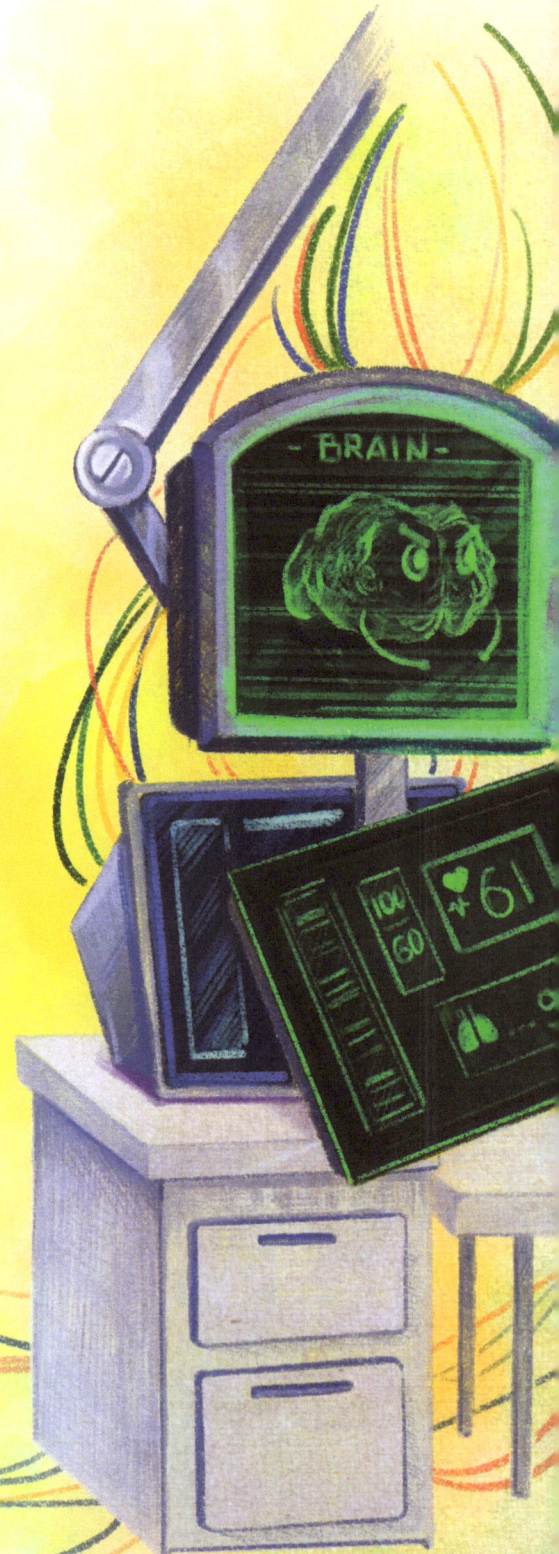

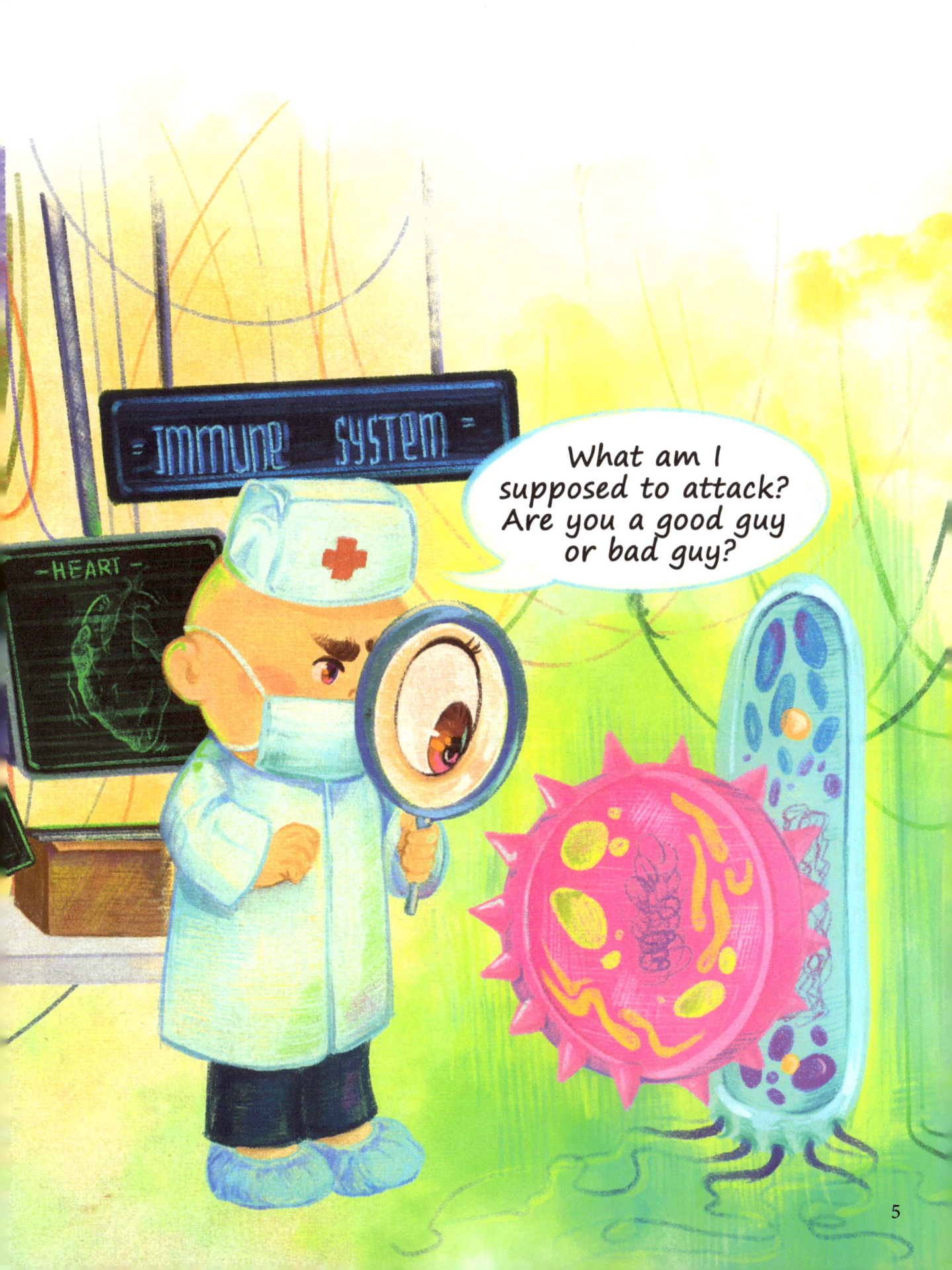

Really cool kids with PANS/PANDAS might...

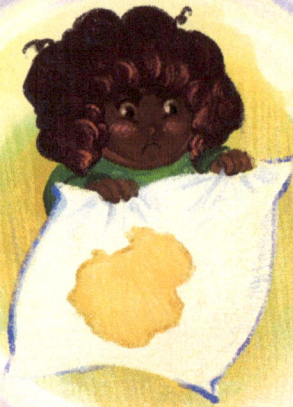

... have sleep problems (bad dreams, or trouble falling or staying asleep);

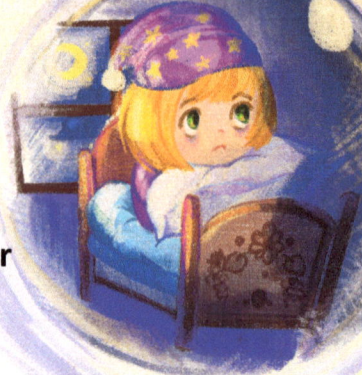

... need to pee more often, or start wetting the bed (wearing pull-ups until your body figures it out might help);

... develop odd movements ("tics"); handwriting, drawing and coordination might get worse;

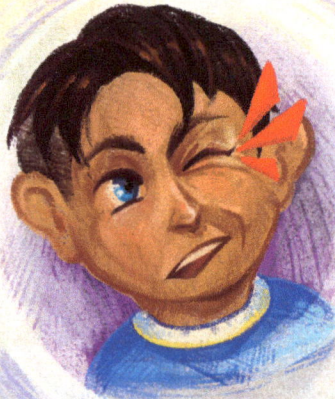

Parents can help

Recognize that *none* of this is "on purpose." Meet your child's needs based on how they are feeling and behaving today.

- Are they acting younger?
- Are they exhibiting new behaviors?
- Do they have new fears?

Provide comfort, support, and structure based on what your child is currently capable of.

Talk to your care team. Remember – overcoming adversity builds resilience.

... feel really, really anxious, depressed, angry, or have SOOO MANY FEELINGS they overflow;

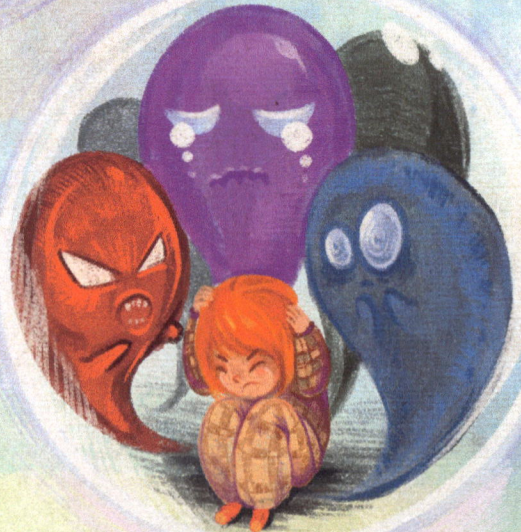

... get unusual ideas about food (and stop eating certain foods);

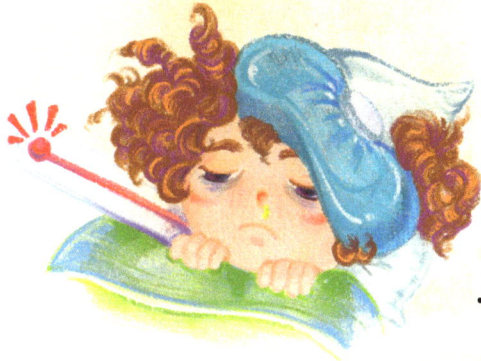

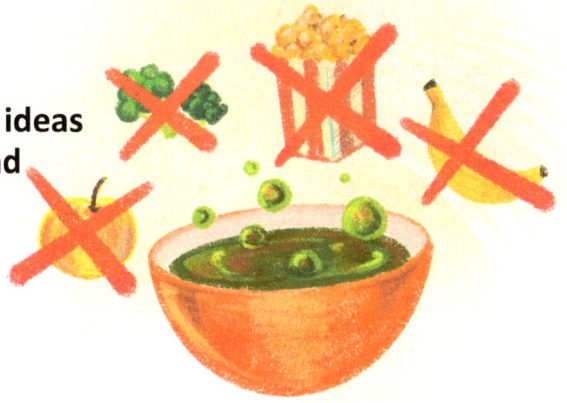

... have fevers;

... have a really hard time focusing, thinking, and problem solving

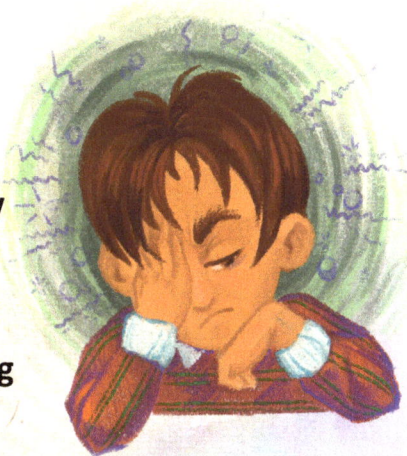

... feel younger than they are, and do things a younger child would; or

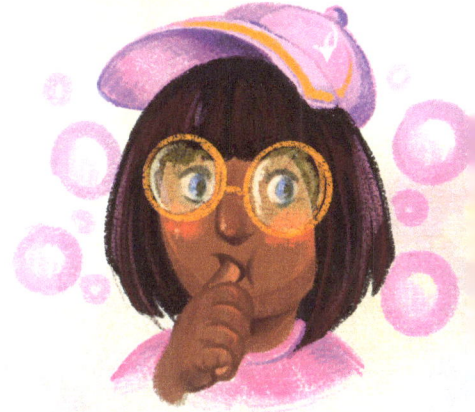

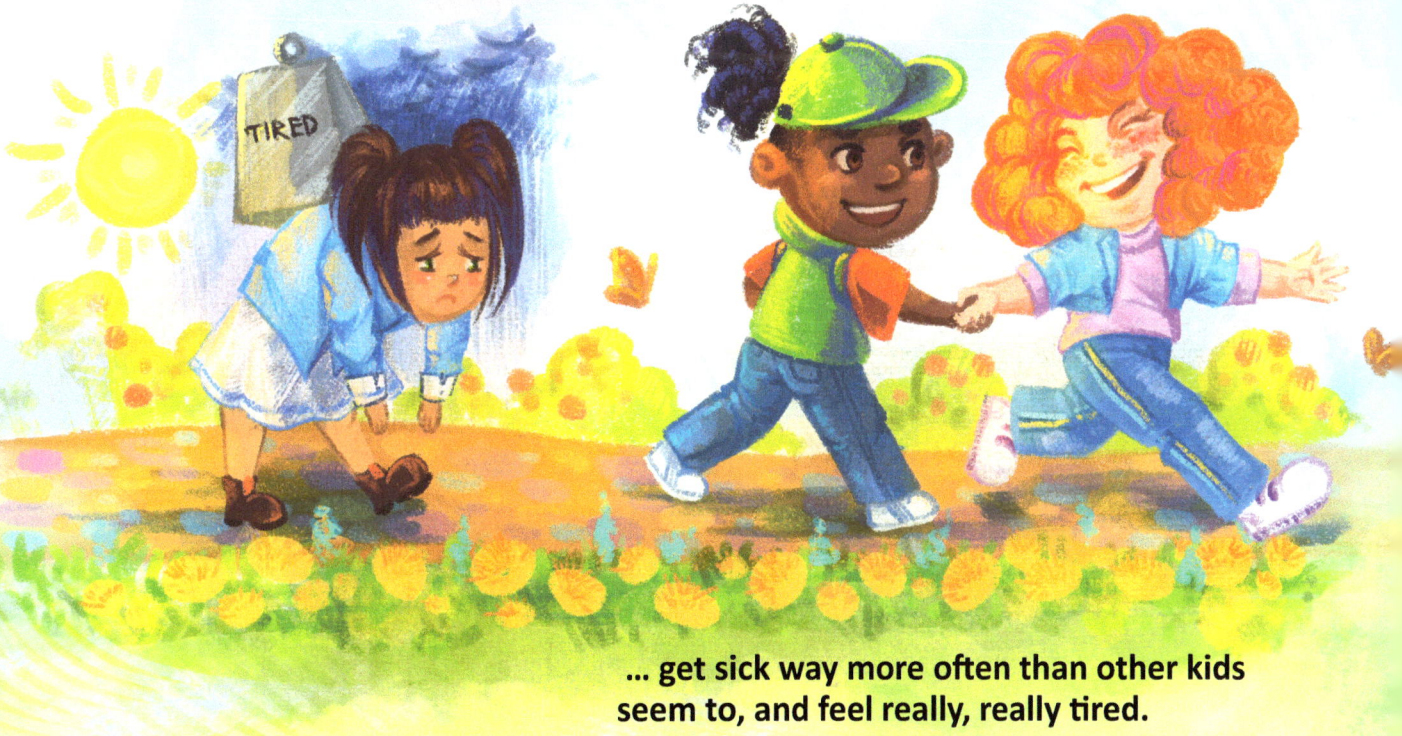

... get sick way more often than other kids seem to, and feel really, really tired.

Doctors are detectives

If you are sick and don't get well within a day or two, you might go to your family doctor in a clinic, or to the hospital. It is your doctor's job to figure out what is wrong, and *how to help your body get healthy.*

Doctors work with other health care professionals. Everyone wants to figure out how to help you feel better.

You are part of the healthcare team. It is your body that does the challenging work of getting you well. You have the most important job!

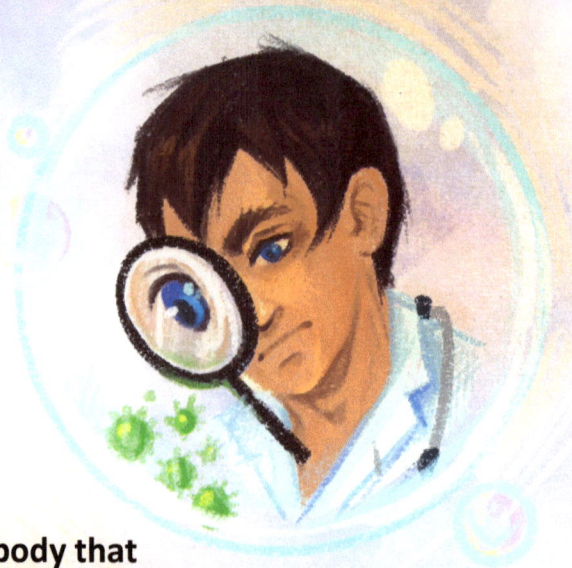

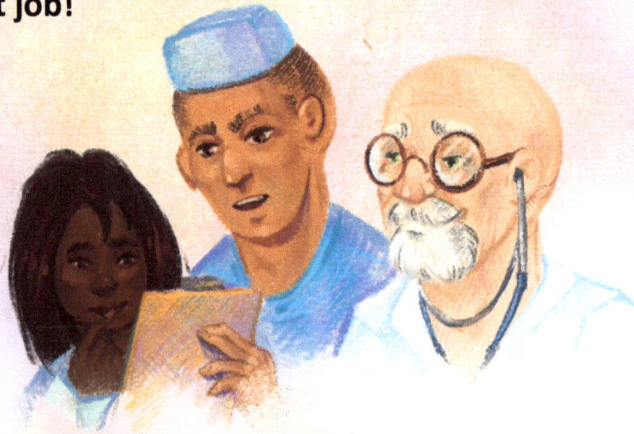

What does your doctor and treatment team do to figure out what is going on?

Let's talk about it. Here are some things that might happen:

The team will talk to you and your family.

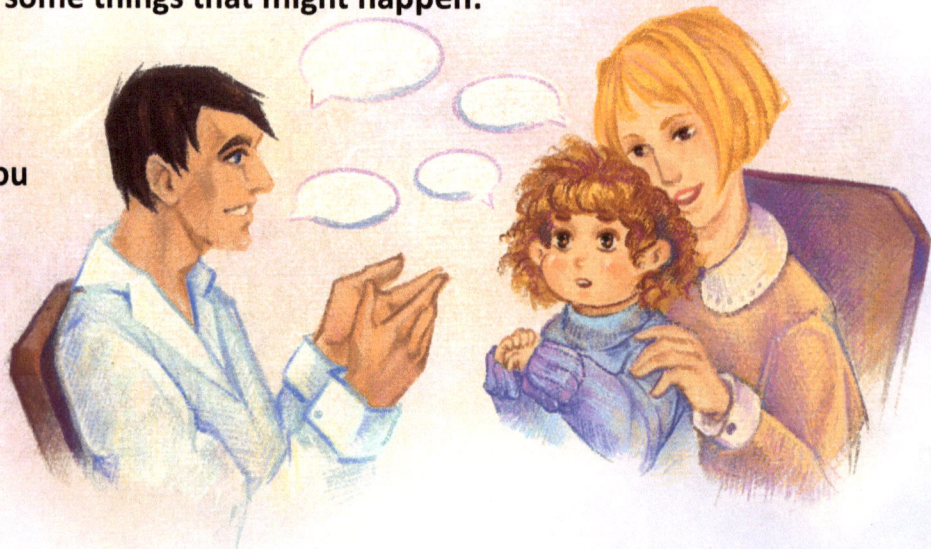

They might take your temperature,

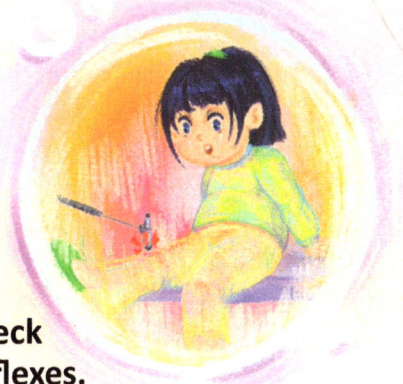

listen to your chest,

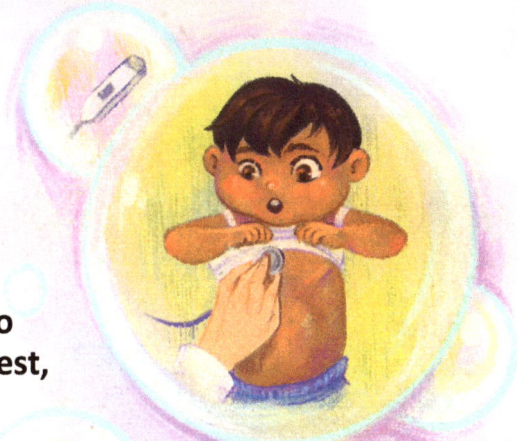

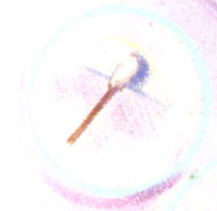

and check your reflexes.

They might use cotton swabs to take samples from inside your nose and throat, and collect blood samples.

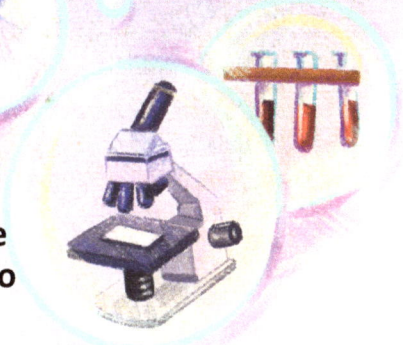

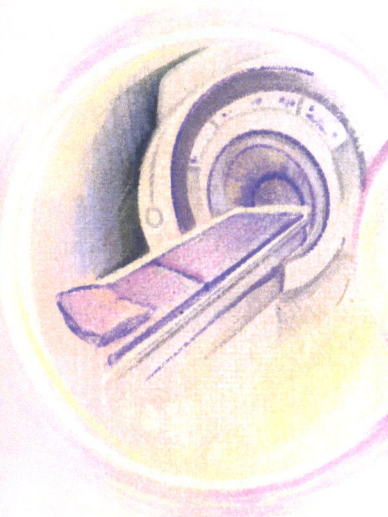

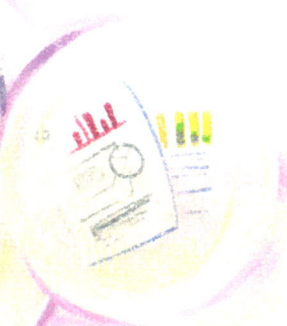

They might take images (pictures), like x-rays.

They might monitor your sleep.

They will do LOTS of paperwork.

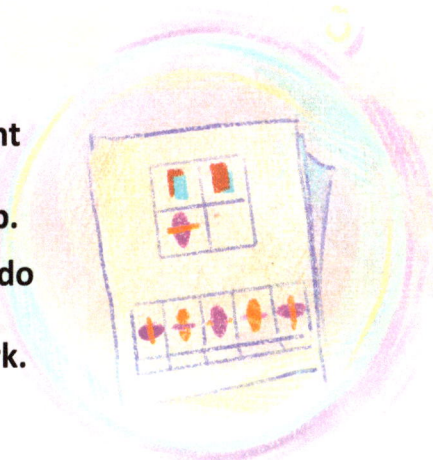

You need to know

There is no "one" test to rule PANS/PANDAS in or out.

You may feel overwhelmed.

Pick an affirmation and use it often. Some examples:

- I can do this.
- I am strong, and brave.
- I can get through one thing at a time.
- I am capable.

Mom and Dad can help you find an affirmation. They need one too!

Uh-oh. It IS *PANS/PANDAS!*

The doctors have run all their tests, ruled everything else out, and have diagnosed PANS/PANDAS.

Now what?

Parents can help

If your child has PANS/PANDAS your job includes:

- ✓ Educating yourself.

- ✓ Keeping your child safe at home, or in the hospital if needed. Abrupt psychiatric symptoms may cause safety concerns.

- ✓ Changing your own expectations daily, to match what your child is capable of moment by moment.

- ✓ Maintaining your child's self-esteem. Increase positive validation for specific "wins," even if it is for something they did well a year ago.

Your child's best will be different daily.

Your child will have lots of different feelings, and may have big behavioral changes. Behavioral and emotional regression usually happens with PANS/PANDAS. Shaming, blaming, and anger do NOT help. Your child needs unconditional love, support, and encouragement.

Empower your child. Encourage self-reliance in all the little things, while you increase your level of care to meet their needs.

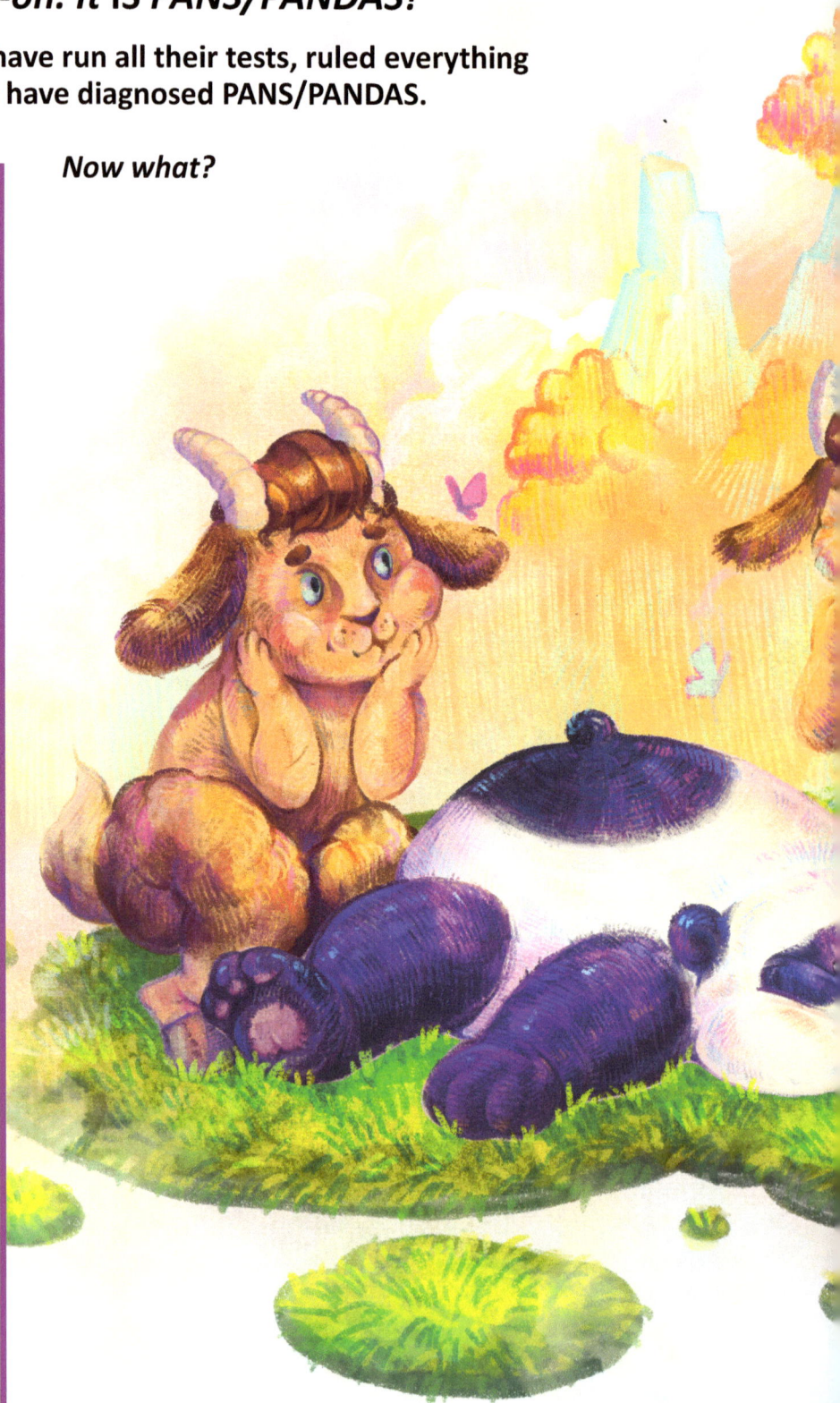

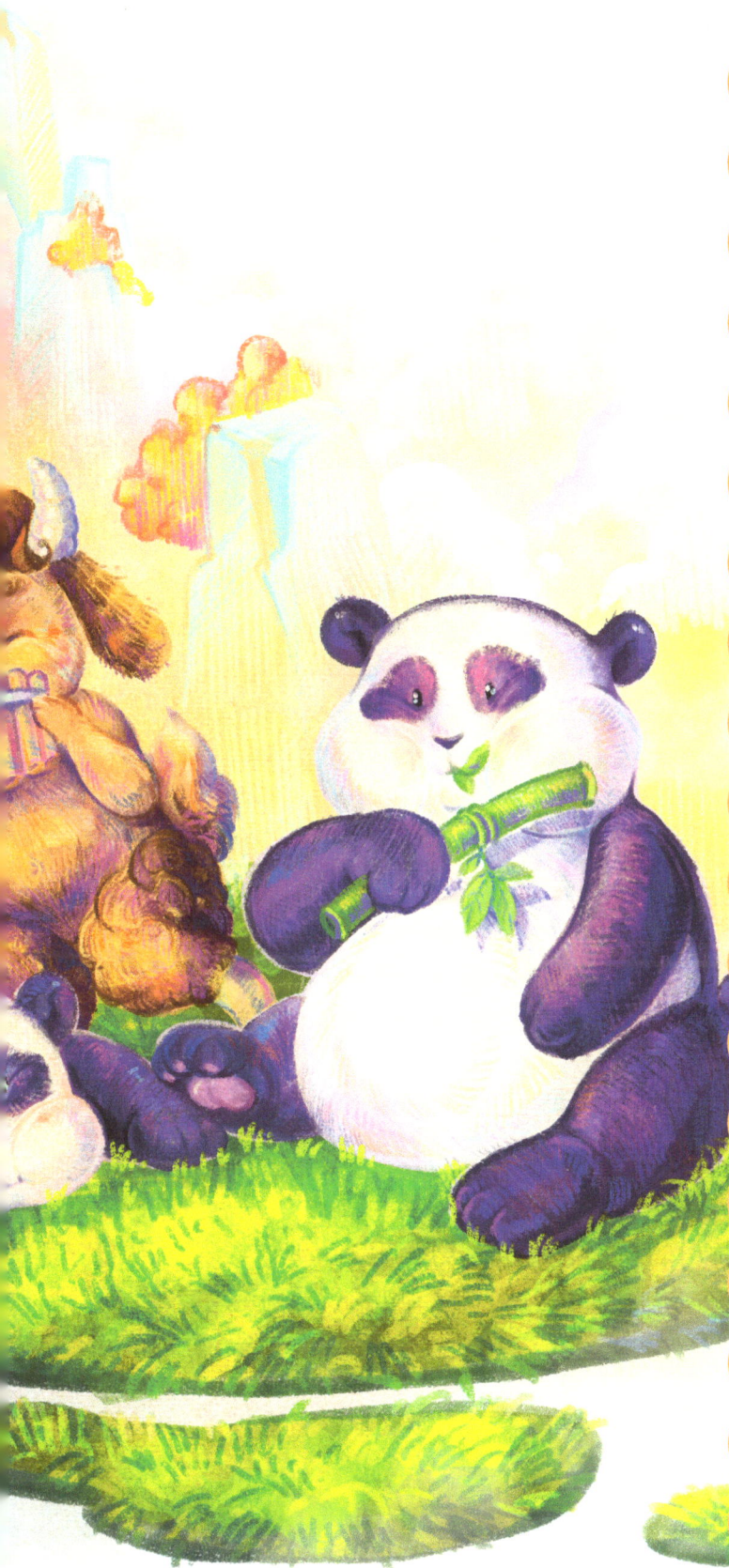

Tasks: These are for you, kiddo!

It is your job to make choices about the many things you can! (There will be choices you don't get to make.)

- Do you want orange leggings or blue pants today?

- Do you want mac and cheese or hotdogs for supper?

- Would you prefer your left arm or right arm for bloodwork?

- Do you want a blueberry or strawberry smoothie after the doctor's office?

- Do you need a quiet time to reset? (If yes, ask!)

Tell your parents AND your care team how you feel.

Take a breath, and think before you speak. When you can, be clear and use your words to describe your thoughts, feelings and behaviors.

Sometimes we cry if we are upset. That is okay too. Feeling afraid or upset, AND being brave, go together. Ask for a hug!

You are growing and changing every day. That is part of being a kid. When you have PANS/PANDAS, things can change in ways we don't like. If you are sick, it is even more important to communicate well.

11

What should I expect?

Having PANS/PANDAS can feel like being on a roller coaster.

It can be a single episode (you get sick once and get better).

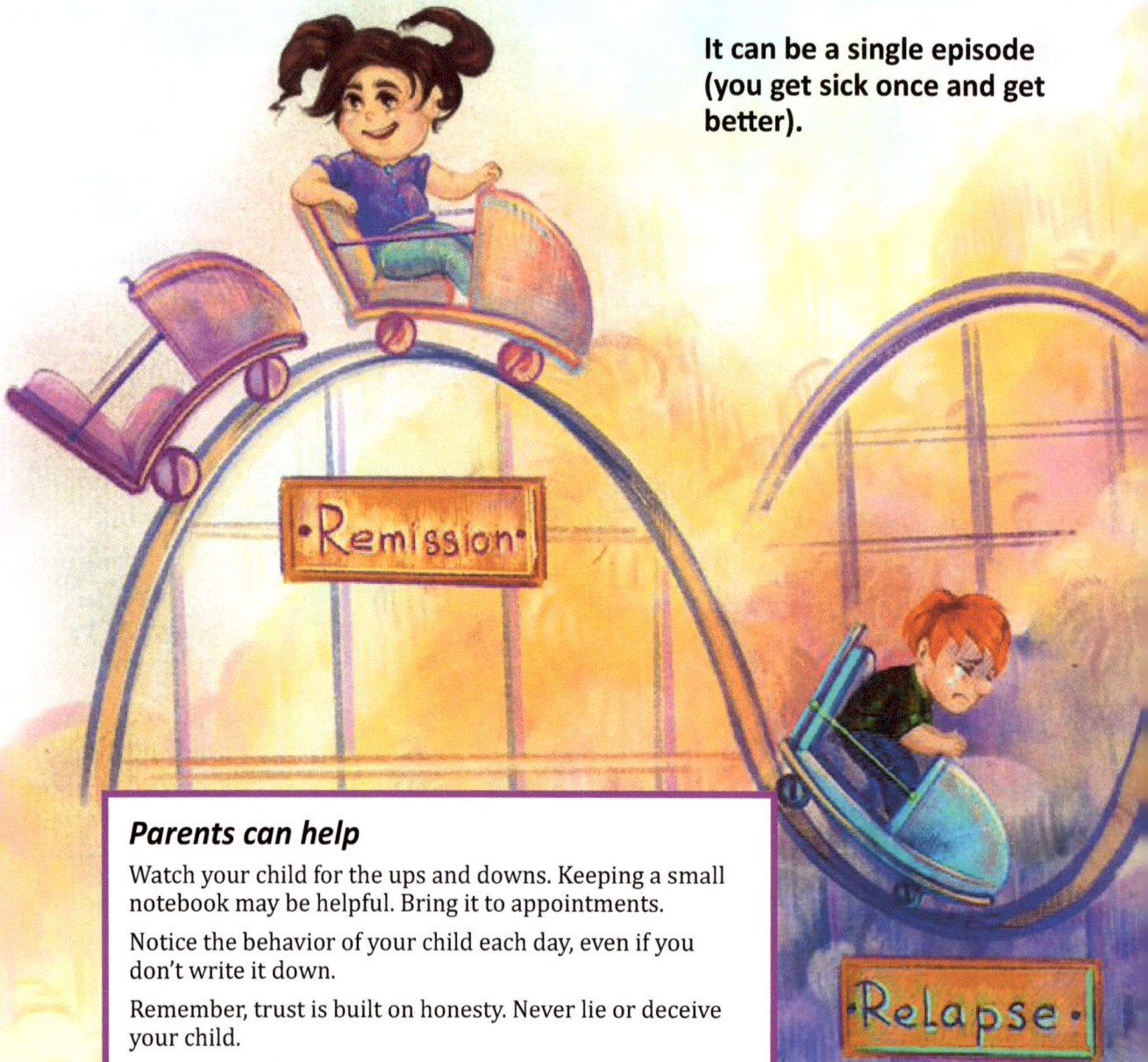

Remission

Relapse

Parents can help

Watch your child for the ups and downs. Keeping a small notebook may be helpful. Bring it to appointments.

Notice the behavior of your child each day, even if you don't write it down.

Remember, trust is built on honesty. Never lie or deceive your child.

Tell them the truth. Instead of saying: "Sit still while they take your blood," it is more helpful to say: "It will hurt a little bit. Will you be brave?"

Be the best caregiver you can be.

Or, it can be chronic, with *relapses* (you have symptoms again) and *remissions* (you feel better).

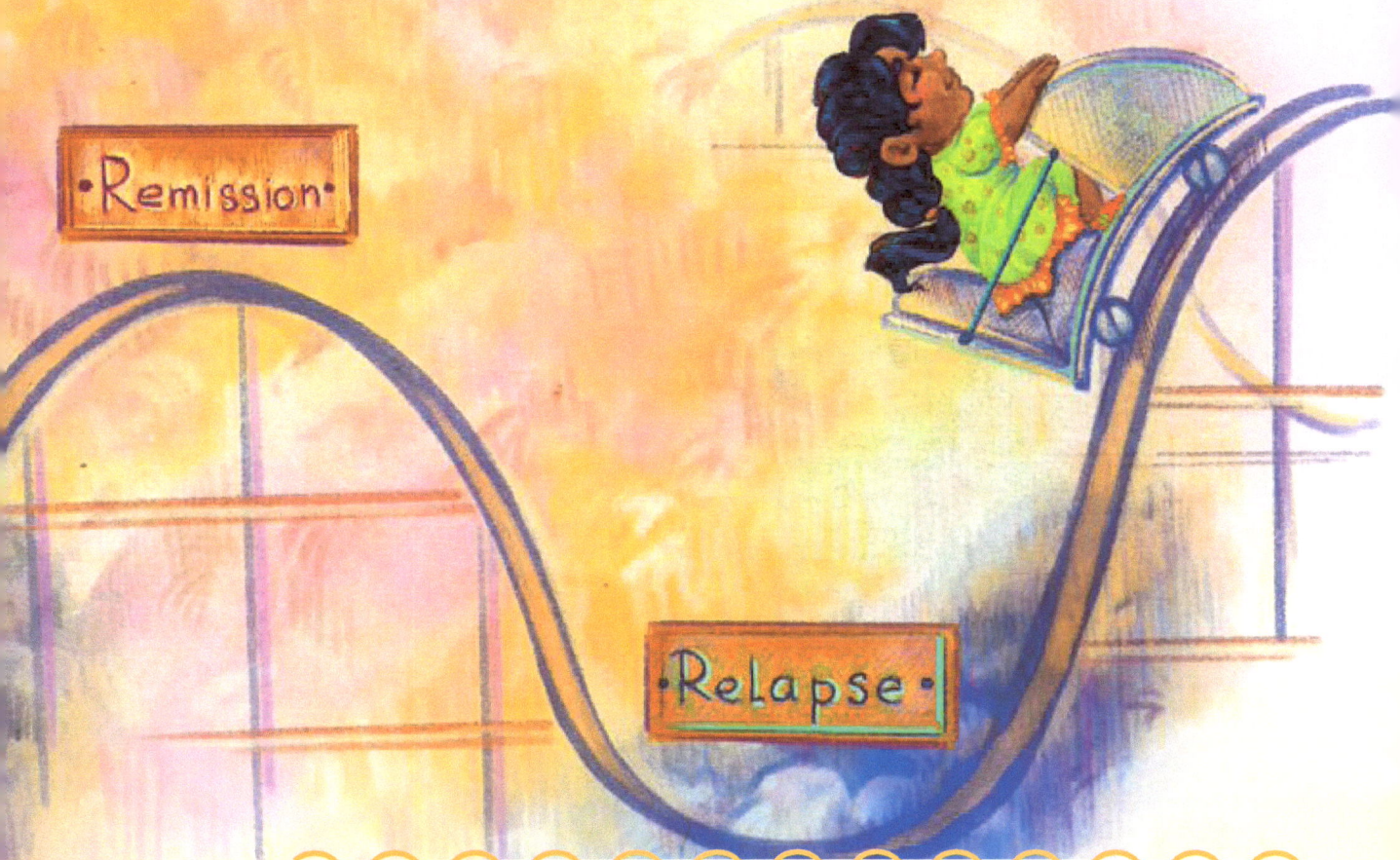

·Remission·

·Relapse·

What you can do

It is easy to feel discouraged when you have a relapse, and super excited on a day you feel better. Learn to take things one day at a time. Say: "I will do my best based on how I feel today."

Is my immune system struggling, too?

80% of kids with PANS/PANDAS have immune system problems.

Your immune system has a job to do.

It recognizes germs or viruses, and sends soldier cells to fight the infections.

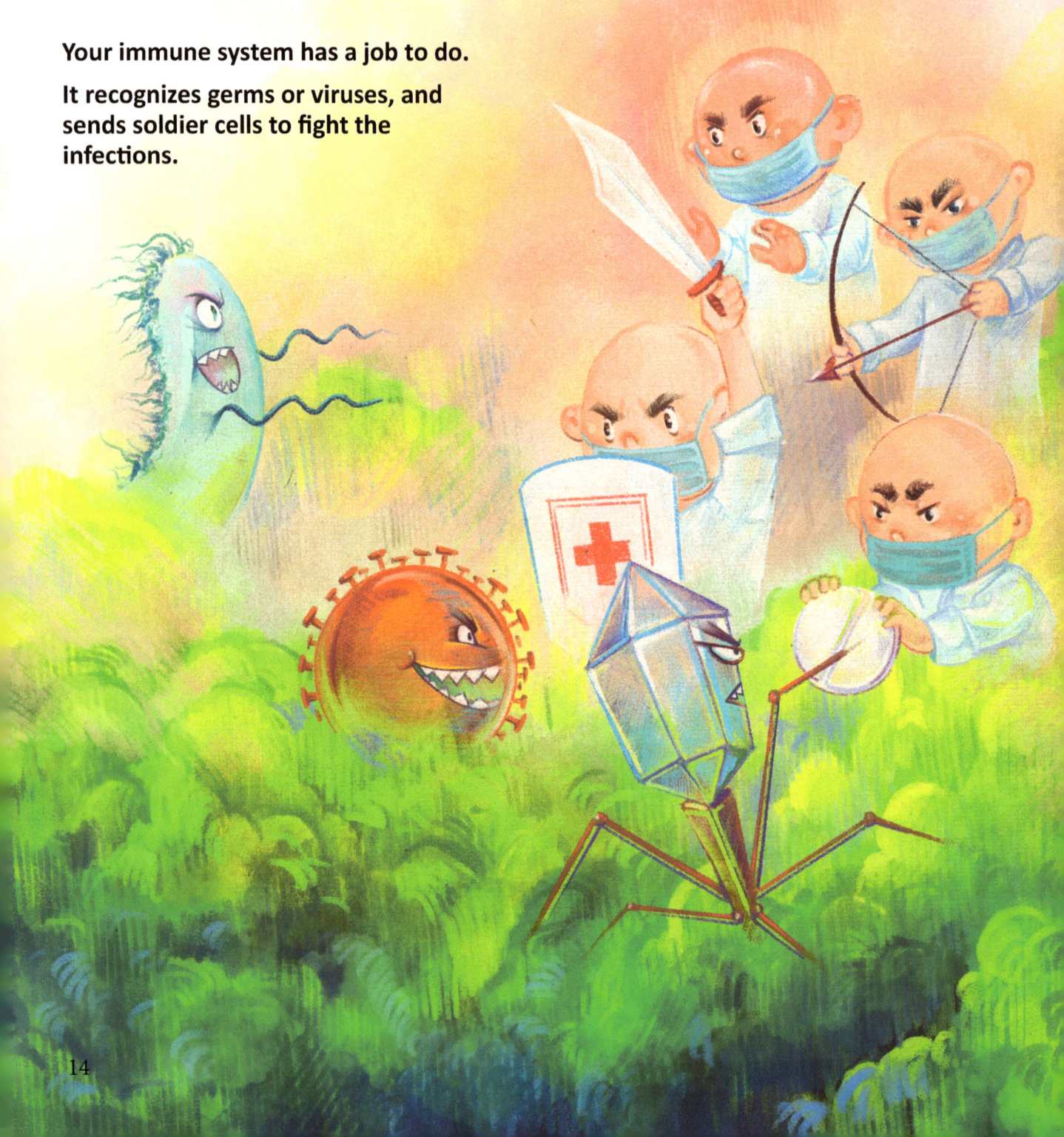

When you have PANS/PANDAS, the immune system gets confused. Sometimes it attacks your own body!

This is an *autoimmune response.*

immunity

Sometimes your immune system is not strong enough to fight infections.

This means you are *immunocompromised,* and need to avoid infection if you can.

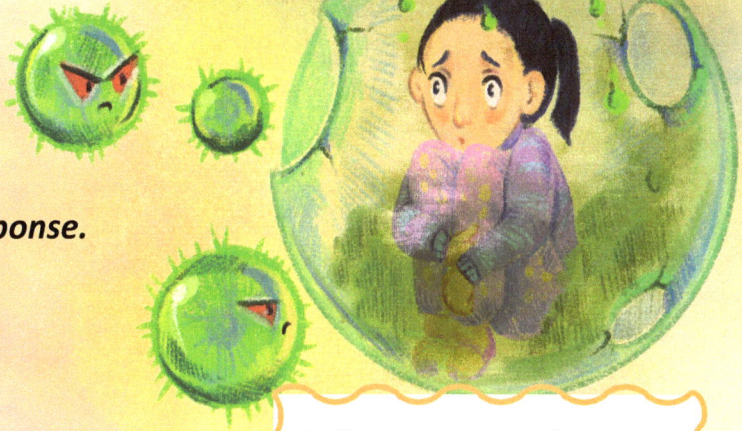

What you can do to help yourself

- Stay away from sick people.
- Wash your hands.
- Use hand sanitizer.
- Wear a mask if your doctor tells you to.
- Play outside if the weather is nice.
- Get enough rest to support your body.

You might also need medication, supplements and a healthy diet to help your immune system. It could be a pill or it could be medicine that needs to go into your vein with a tiny IV. It is like a superpower going into you.

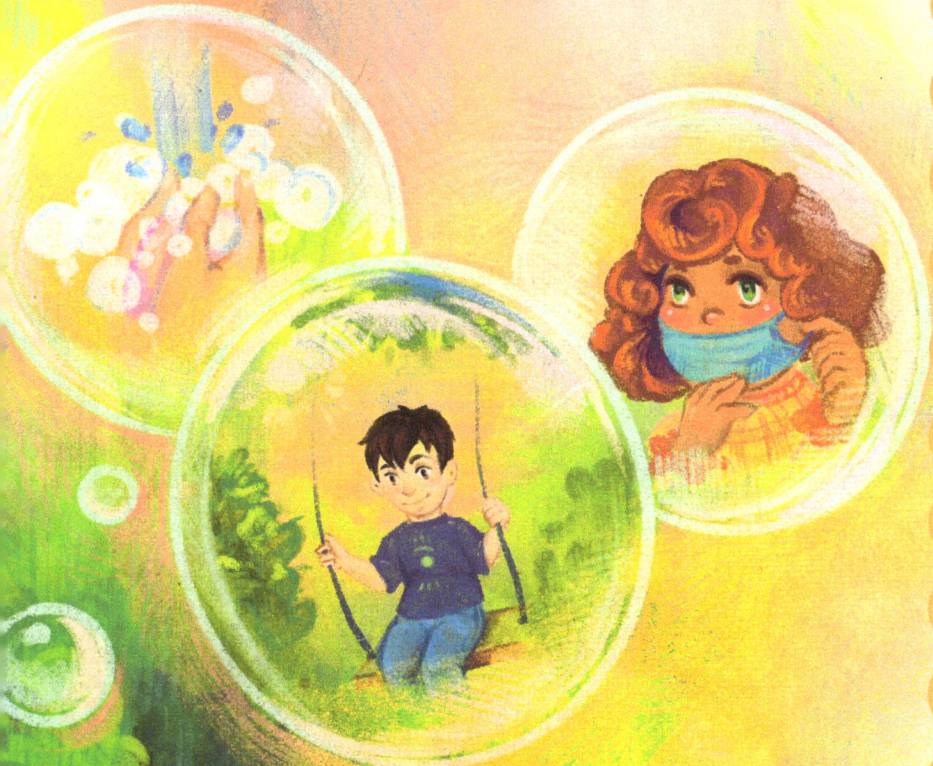

15

What about at school?

With PANS/PANDAS your brain struggles with focus, concentration, and feeling foggy. You might have headaches, or have difficulty with handwriting, sitting still, or doing things the way you used to.

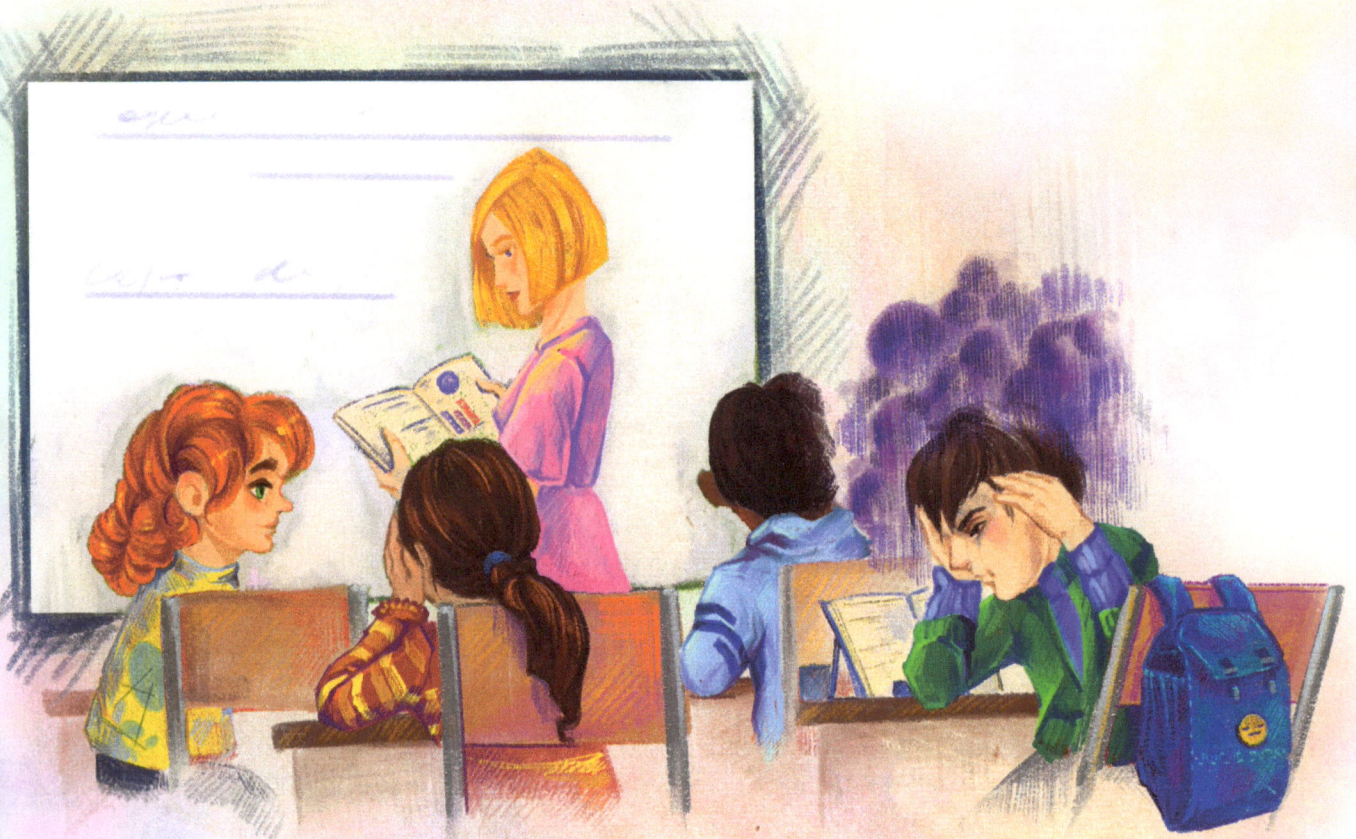

Teachers and parents can help

A child diagnosed with PANS/PANDAS requires an individualized education plan (I.E.P.) to adjust expectations and take the pressure off. Schoolwork and homework may take more time, require one-to-one support, and need to be broken into smaller/shorter chunks.

Make a safe place in the classroom where the child can go for a 20-30 minute "reboot," and empower them to make choices about what they need. Remember, this timeout place is not punitive, but supportive.

A child with PANS/PANDAS may benefit from a study-buddy.

When a child with PANS/PANDAS misses school, make getting back on track more manageable. Decrease homework, add more breaks and scheduled rests.

Your teacher, the school psychologist and your parents will come up with a plan to help you.

Your job is to tell them what you feel and think.

Do your best, and get back on track if things go downhill!

Tell them how you feel.

What you can do to help yourself at school

- Use fidget strategies like a spinner or a squeezy ball.

- Doodle.

- Set up a secret signal with your teacher (a touch on the shoulder means "get back on track").

- Run errands for the teacher so you can get up more often.

- "Chunk it." Do one thing at a time until it is done, then go to the next.

- Use sticky notes to get and stay organized.

- Tell your teacher when you need a "reboot." Go to your designated safe space for a time-limited break.

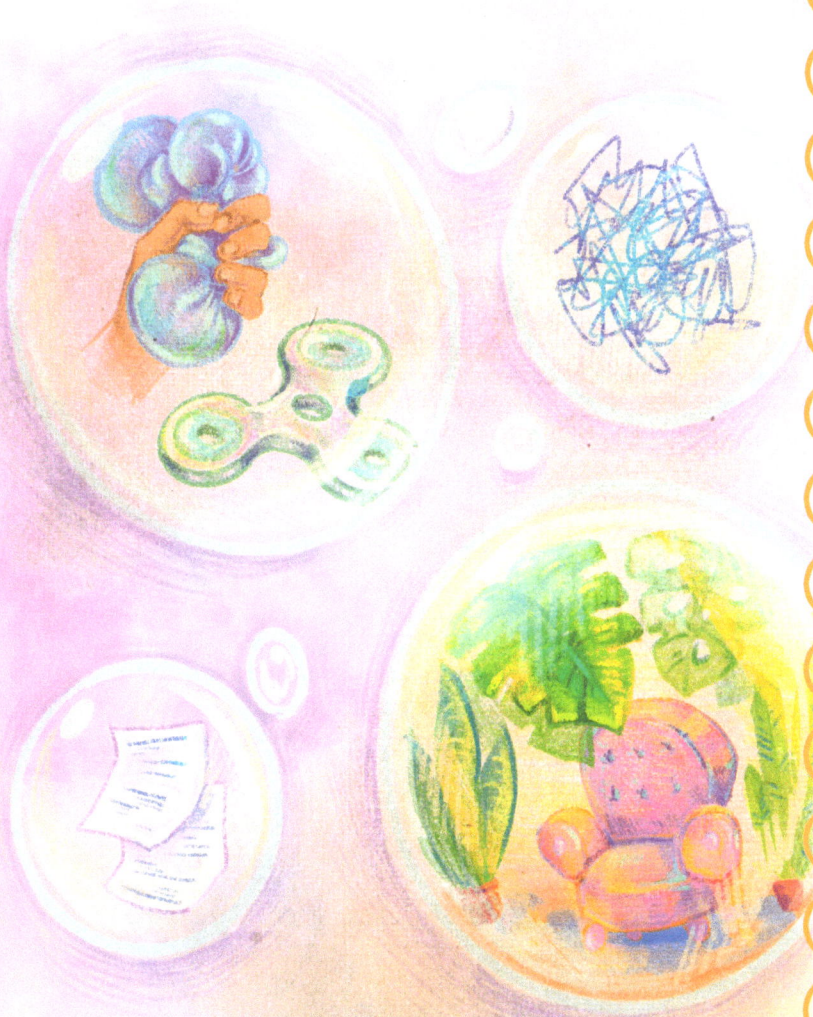

What if I'm having trouble sleeping?

You might have sleep problems, like feeling anxious and scared, or having bad dreams and nightmares. Some kids with PANS/PANDAS have problems waking up enough to pee at night, too.

Parents can help

Separation anxiety, bed-wetting and sleep issues are common with PANS/PANDAS. It may seem as though your child is younger than before. New fears show up, new obsessions, and new symptoms. Shaming, blaming and anger won't help. The feelings are real to your child.

How can you help? There is no "one right answer" that works for everyone.

For nightmares, try giving extra cuddles or other non-verbal comfort until they can talk about it. Lay down with them for a while. Tell them "You are safe. It was a dream and not real." Stay calm and comforting—no anger, even if you are tired.

For bed-wetting, get a mattress protector. Have extra sheets in the bedroom, and be matter of fact as you change the bed without criticism. If needed, help your child have a quick bath and change their pajamas, and tuck them back in. Using pull-ups can help a lot, too. Remind your child to pee before bed. Talk to the doctor and/or psychologist for other suggestions.

If separation anxiety reappears, try whatever worked when your child was going through this before. While your child is really struggling, it may be easier to go to them ten times a night (if you need your bedroom to be child free), or you may prefer to put a mattress on your floor.

Do what works for your family. You know your child best. Problem solve with them.

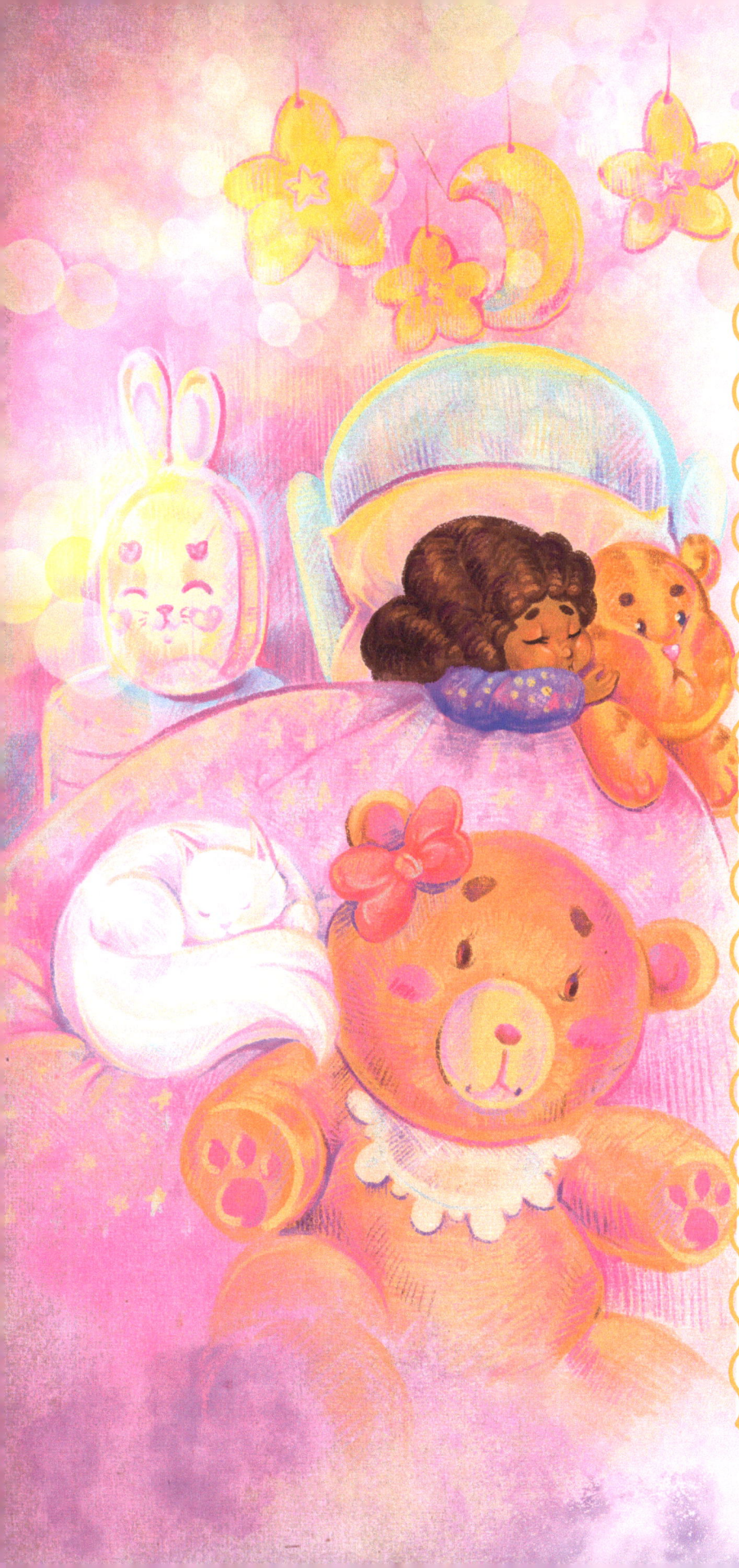

What you can do to help yourself sleep better

Even little choices can help. Before bed, think:

- Would I like a nightlight or small lamp?

- Would I like the door open or closed?

- Would I like to listen to soothing music, or an audiobook of a favorite story?

- Would I like an extra hug?

- Would I like to be tucked in, snug as a bug – or have loose bed covers?

Making these choices helps you feel in control.

Routines help you relax. For example, each evening have a relaxing bath, listen to a story, and get tucked in.

Make your bed a happy zone, with cozy pajamas and bedding, stuffed animals, a pet (if you have one), and happy colors.

Sometimes my emotions feel out of control!

Our brain helps us think. It also helps us manage our moods through *neurotransmitters* – little messengers that keep our feelings in an "okay" zone.

With PANS/PANDAS, emotions can get very big and chaotic (all jumbled and changing quickly). You may feel very anxious, very depressed, very angry, or ALL of them at once.

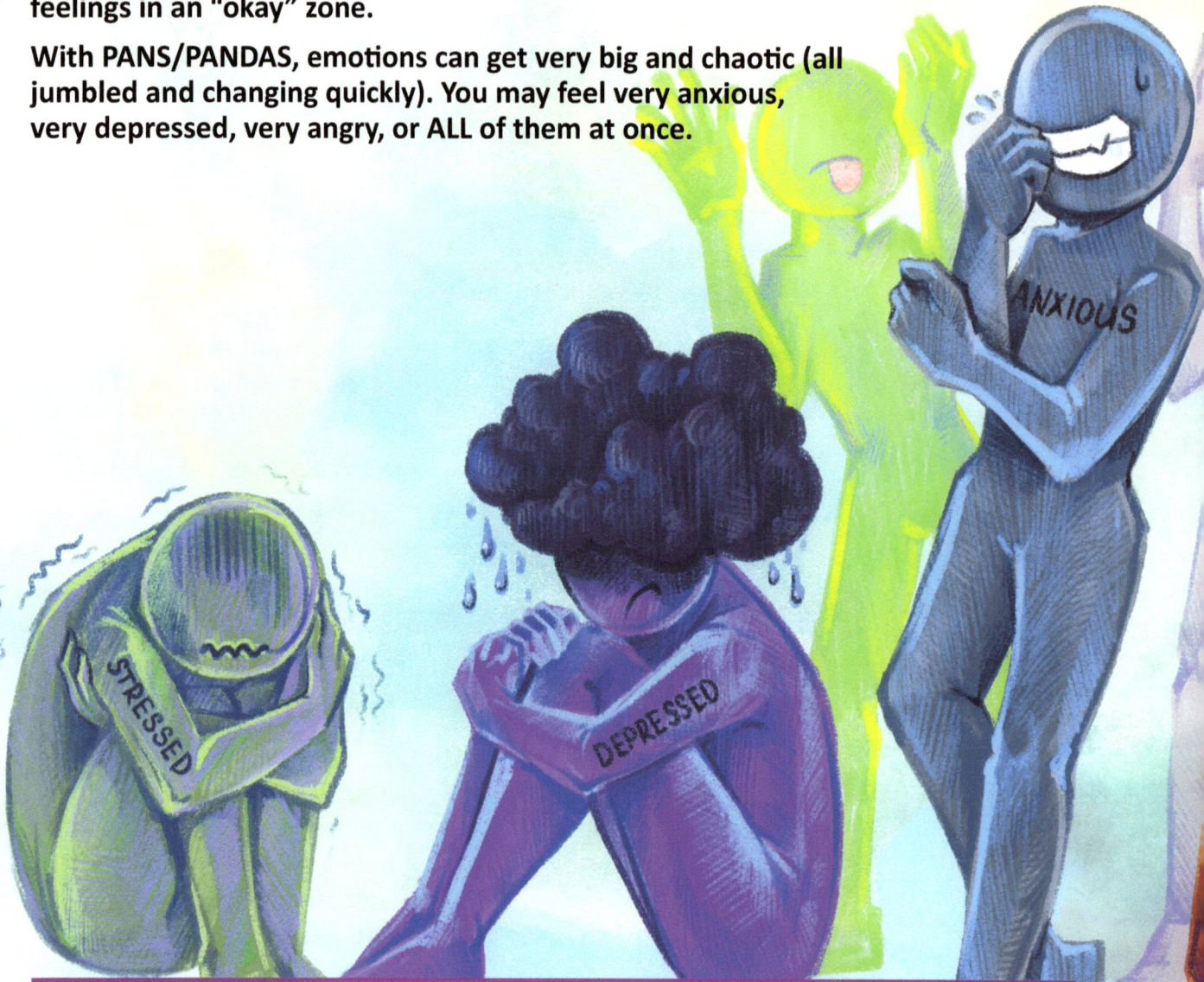

Parents can help

Help your child with mood regulation. Move your child to an area or situation with less stimulation (quieter, fewer people, less chaotic).

Teach a stress pause – slow down a situation, encourage control – "If you are upset count to ten, then answer. Stop, think, and chill."

Teach calming breaths: Sit cross-legged, soften your belly, breathe in slowly through your nose with longer, slower exhales through your mouth. Do it with your child. Count if it helps them.

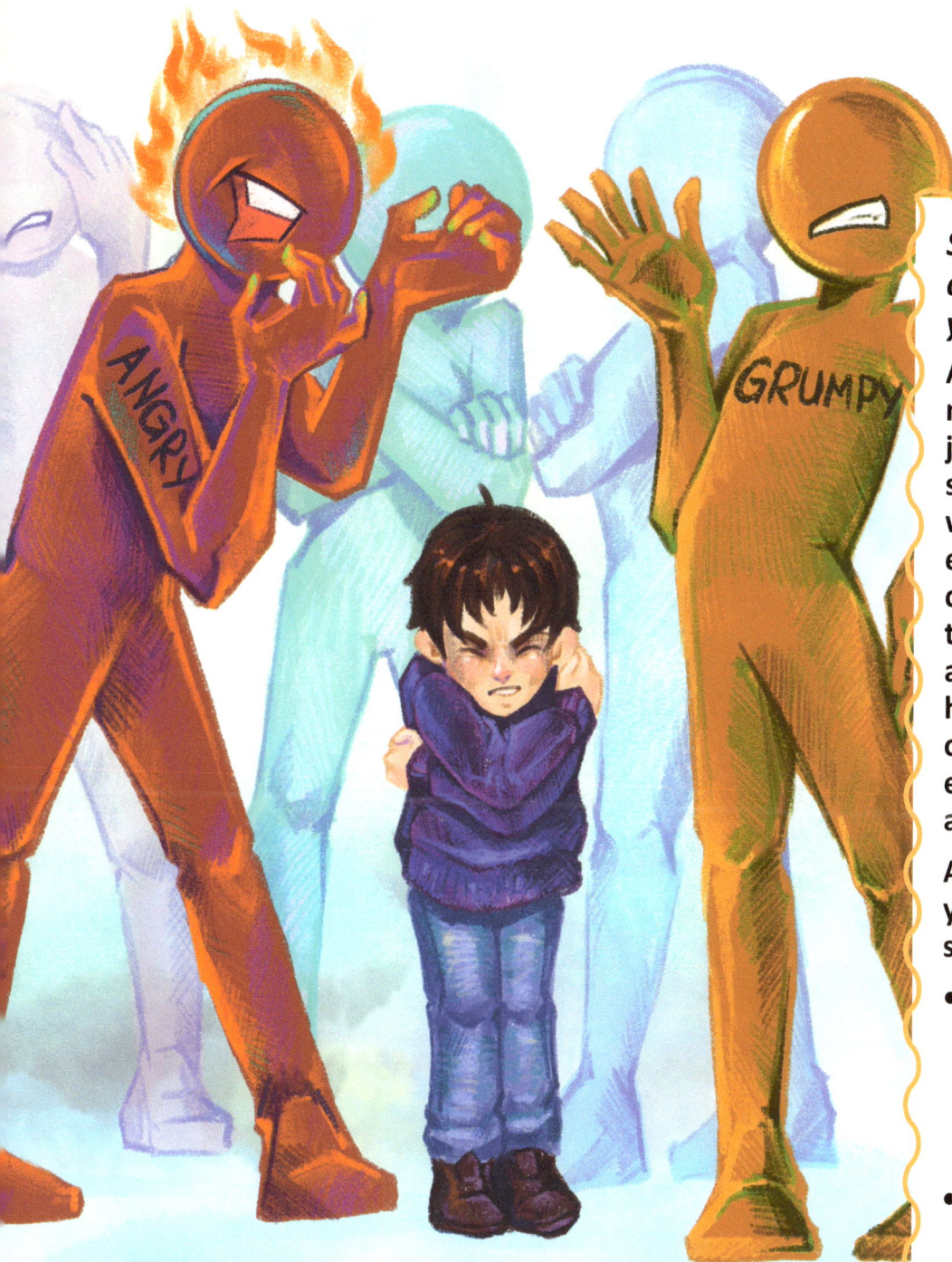

Strategies you can use to help yourself

All emotions are normal. They just get "BIG" sometimes. How we express big emotions is what can get us into trouble, so we all have to learn how to control our attention, emotions, thoughts and actions.

Adults will help you practice these strategies:

- Share feelings in a safe way: "I didn't sleep much so I am grumpy."

- Label your emotions. Giving how you feel a name can help you take control.

Humorous ENRICHED *Elusive* Easy-going Insulted Gracious

FRIGHTENED Careless Kindhearted **Afraid** Jittery

Terrified Critical **Abrasive** Effective Alert **Afraid** Jittery

Intrigued **Great** *Cuddly* *dazzling* **Fidgety** *Lability* Frustrated

Generous *Embarrassed* *elite* Absurd ADVENTUROUS

COURAGEOUS Lost *magical* **Gloomy** *Committed*

Disrespected EMPHATIC Coy FEROCIOUS Flexible

Astounded Ignored Jubilant HESITANT Hated

Challenged BOTHERED *Amorous*

Agreeable INTENSE Acknowledged **Miserable**

Gleeful *Attractive* HORRENDOUS Keen Enabled

Cold-hearted Encouraged *Hysterical*

Gusty **Bossy** *Delighted* **Admired** Timid *Homely*

Introverted JAUNTY IRATE *Manipulated* *mean*

Gentle Cowardly **Disconnected** Suspicious

HOSTILE Absorbed Bitter Merry mighty

Fragile ESSENTIAL *Absent-minded* **Disgusting** *Accepted*

Haughty **Insistent** EXUBERANT Lonesome **Forlorn**

What am I <u>feeling</u>?

22

INTIMIDATED GRUMPY ABANDONED. Happy-go-lucky Deceptive Eloquent emotional

Impish FRIENDLY HATEFUL Festive DEPRESSED ASSERTIVE Cheerful

Dependable determined Imaginative EDGY Discriminated Enchanted CHIVALROUS

Bored ANGRY ANNOYED ABRUPT Creative Healthy Impatient Feisty Fortunate

Content Dejected Childlike clever Conscientious Jovial ALONE Appalled argumentative

Mediocre Bullied Loving Idealistic ABYSMAL Abusive Mellow CONCERNED

Betrayed Crazy Aggressive ambivalent LOATHSOME Overjoyed Doubtful Innocent

Compatible Deceived Elegant DEDICATED Melancholy Blissful Messy Adrift

Heard Competent Fascinated Important Calm Faint hearted Joyful

Humble Homesick Sulky Curious FOOLISH Honest Discouraged

Elated JUSTIFIED Hormonal Faithful Docile DISLIKED

Guarded Brilliant Gullible Careless Envious Amused

Insensitive ENGROSSED Attentive Broken-hearted Adored

Bratty Energetic Helpful Deserving Helpless

Frazzled Grief-stricken Laughable

Funny furious Flustered Anxious

ECCENTRIC ALARMED CODDLED Dismayed Fearful

Breathtaking Worried COMPASSIONATE

Fearless Compelled Amazing. Graceful Gorgeous Crabby

What if my brain starts telling me really weird things?

Some kids with PANS/PANDAS struggle with obsessive-compulsive (OC) symptoms.

- **Obsessions are thoughts or worries that repeat *over and over and over and over*.**

- **Compulsions are behaviors that you feel like you *have to do*.**

How do you know if you have OC symptoms?

- **Are you worrying about the same thing over and over?**

- **Are you repeating behaviors for no reason?**

- **Are you avoiding touching something, even though it isn't harmful to touch?**

- **Are you avoiding eating, or only eating in a certain way?**

Your brain might be telling you to open and close your bedroom door five times, or wash your hands again and again – and you might feel crazy or strange for having weird thoughts and compulsions. (Lots of kids with PANS/PANDAS do.)

If these symptoms are happening to you, talk to your caregiver. This is *not* your fault!! Your brain is mixed up, and is telling you to worry about things that are safe (like eating certain foods), or to do things that are unhealthy choices (like washing your hands until they are raw).

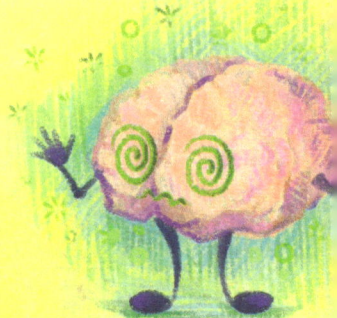

Parents can help

Please don't tell your child to "Just stop it." Obsessions and compulsions are not deliberate, or easily controlled. They are caused by brain changes. Get professional help when you need it. Trust your own instincts. You know your child best.

Tip: Do not give power to the OC symptoms. Characterize/name the symptoms with your child. Do not complete a recurring cycle where you are the rescuer each time. Find a way to change or break the repeating cycle.

- Use phrases such as "Tell 'OC Wonkyness' we are not going to help him."

- Use open-ended questions rather than introducing negatives. "How is your tummy today?" is better than "Does your stomach still hurt like yesterday?"

It is easy to believe it is *always* hard or your child is *always* sick. Put a notebook on the counter. Put a tick each time the repetitive pattern occurs. Keep an objective account of increases and decreases in problematic OC symptoms. ** Note which strategies decrease it (e.g. redirecting, discussing, keeping your child busy with play or stories). This will increase your confidence you have an impact on the situation.

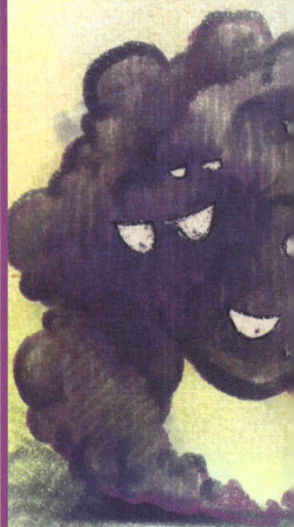

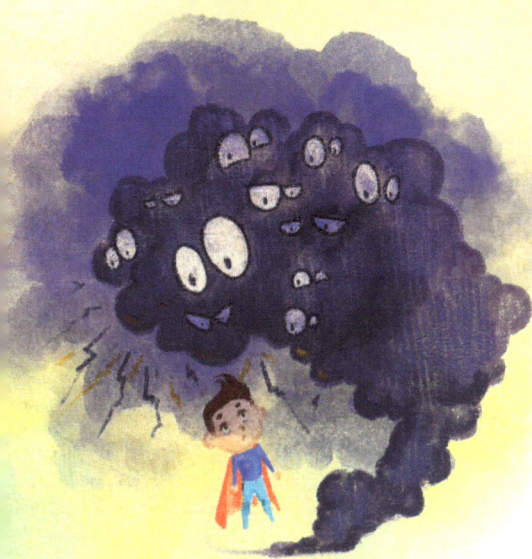

How to tame OC

If you let the OC symptoms be in charge, you might feel less anxious for a minute or two. But the OC symptoms will get bigger, stronger, and more powerful.

You need to learn to be the boss of OC symptoms. Here is a beginning plan!

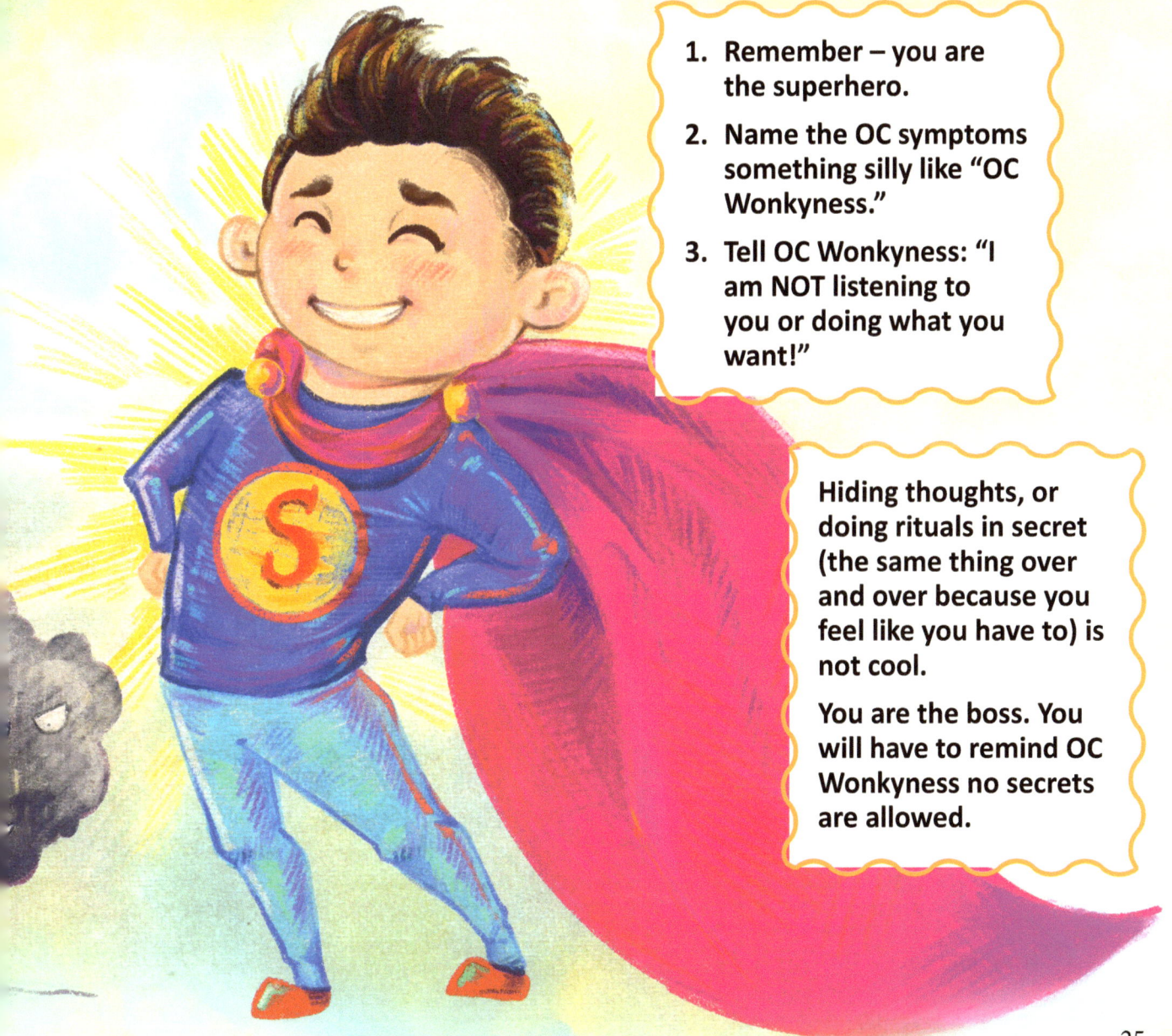

1. Remember – you are the superhero.

2. Name the OC symptoms something silly like "OC Wonkyness."

3. Tell OC Wonkyness: "I am NOT listening to you or doing what you want!"

Hiding thoughts, or doing rituals in secret (the same thing over and over because you feel like you have to) is not cool.

You are the boss. You will have to remind OC Wonkyness no secrets are allowed.

What helps me get healthier?

Time. Sometimes your body, brain and immune system need time to get you healthy.

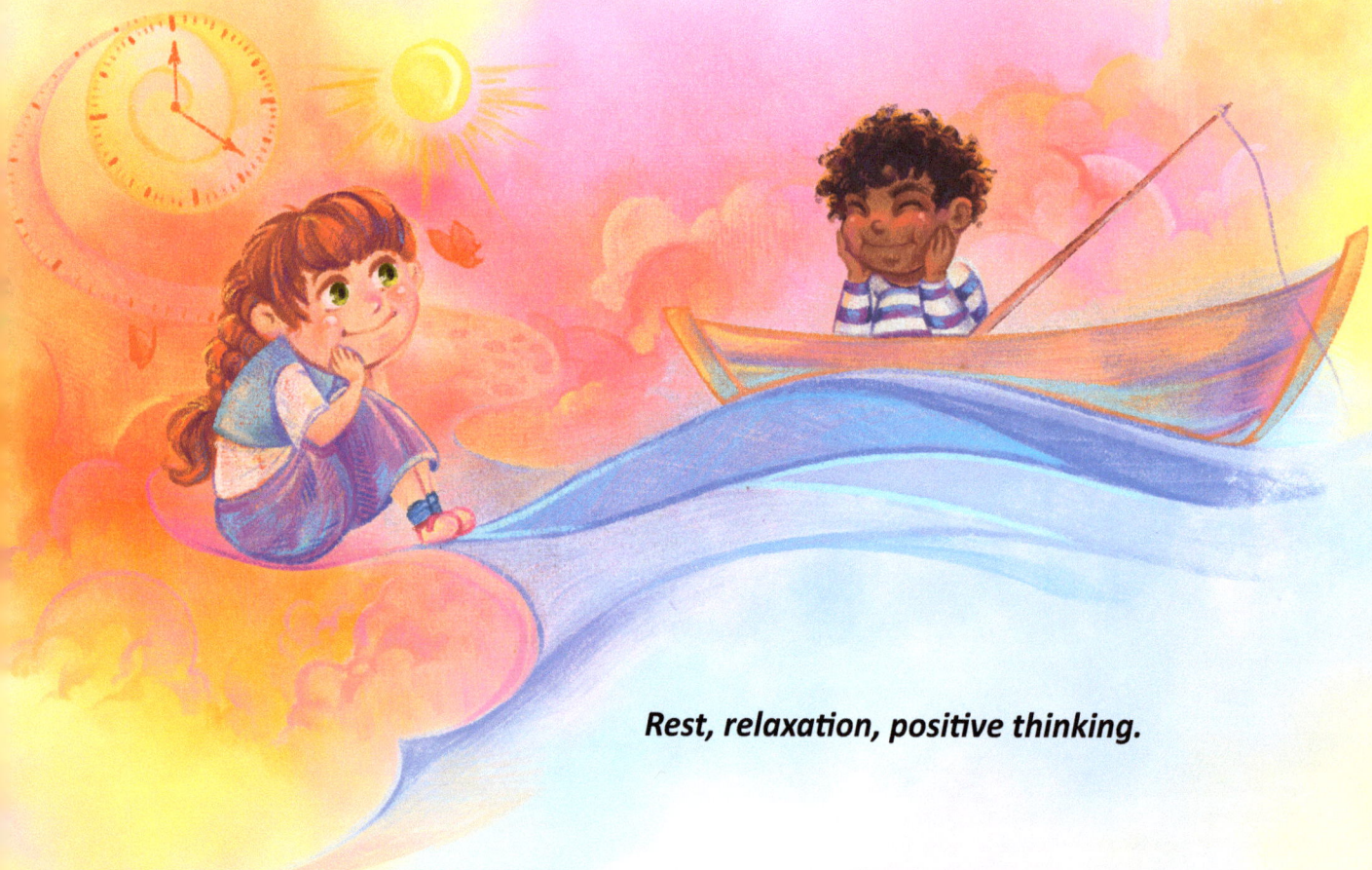

Rest, relaxation, positive thinking.

Parents: Here's what you need to know about your child's medications

The names are long and tough to pronounce, and some sound downright scary.

Take another deep breath, and let it out slowly. You will get through this!

Types of medications:

- Antibiotics, anti-fungals, and antivirals fight bacteria, fungi and viruses.

- Anti-inflammatories (corticosteroids) stop or shorten flares.

- Anti-nausea medication helps when your child feels like they will vomit.

- Mood medications like SSRIs or anti-psychotics help with emotional responses. Remember, this is a physical illness that causes psychiatric issues.

- IMMUNOtherapy (IVIG) supports your child's immune system.

For information about each of the specific medications recommended for your child, talk to your medical team. A pharmacist can help, too.

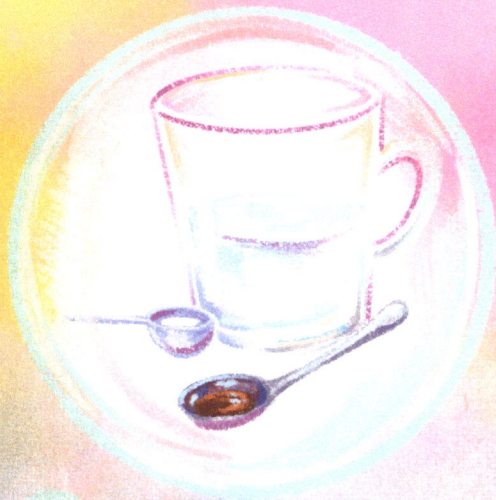

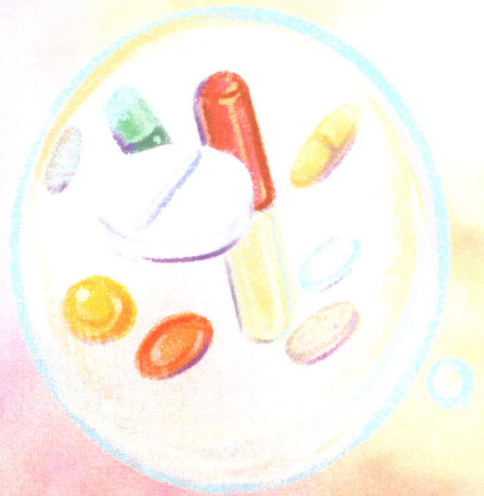

Medications, to fight infection.

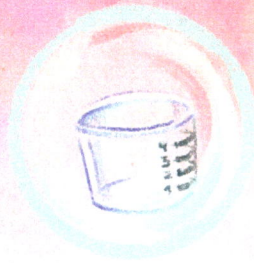

Sometimes the medication to help your immune system needs to go into your vein (IV) through a very tiny needle.

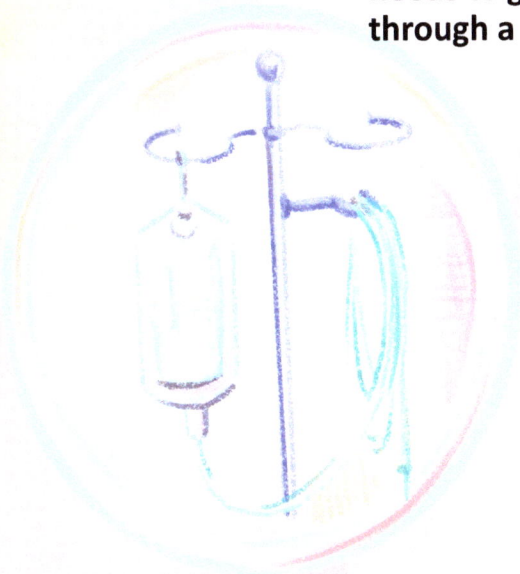

Help make medication work for you

Learn how each medicine works. ASK.

Remember, you are a smart, strong, brave, and capable kid.

How can I avoid (or shorten) flare-ups?

It's helpful to avoid environmental triggers *and* infections. Make choices to support your health.

- Stay away from people who are sick.

- Wash your hands or use sanitizer.

- Wear a mask if your doctor says to.

- Avoid big crowds.

- Sit in a booth or at the edge of a restaurant (not in the middle).

- Keep routines, but be flexible enough to adjust.

- Get enough hours of sleep. Your brain and immune system need rest to stay healthy or recover.

Listen to your body, and learn what you need. When you are super-fatigued, rest *if* it helps, in short, time-limited breaks. ("Restorative" means you feel better when you rest.)

Sometimes with PANS/PANDAS you feel tired no matter what – even if you just woke up, even if it is only halfway through a school day. The best plan is:

- Do one thing at a time. Focus on just that, until it is done.

- Pick again.

How do I feel today?

Parents can help

Emotional stress decreases the immune system's ability to do its job. Remember: Self-confidence develops when kids face obstacles, struggle, and are involved with creating solutions.

Learn to prioritize. Ask yourself, "What is the most important thing to do right now?" Do that.

When you do one thing at a time you are less overwhelmed.

You are the superhero who needs to figure it out.

"I can make my bed."

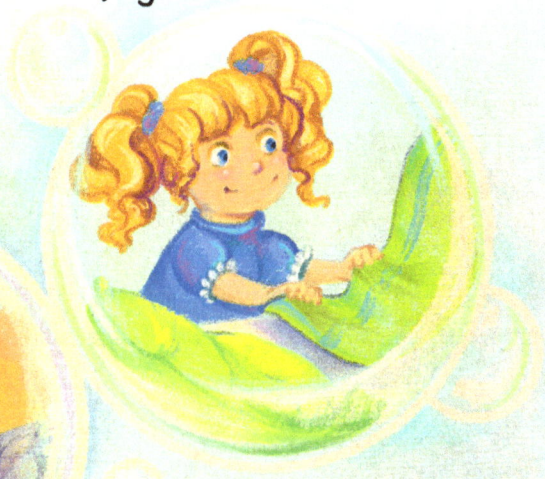

"I can put my pants on."

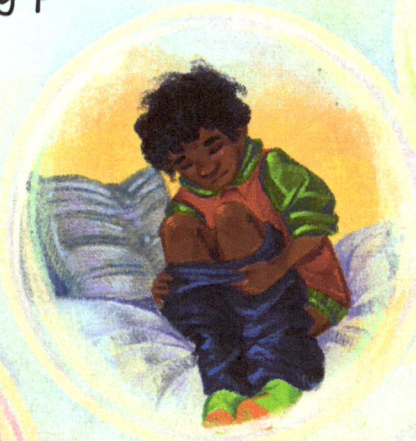

"I can eat three bites of cereal."

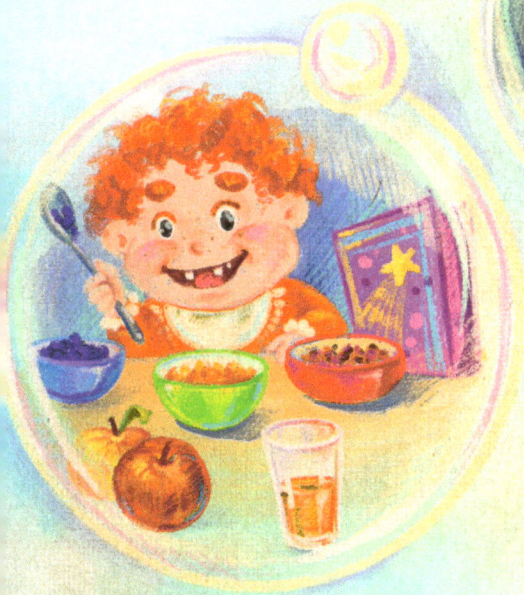

"I need a time out."

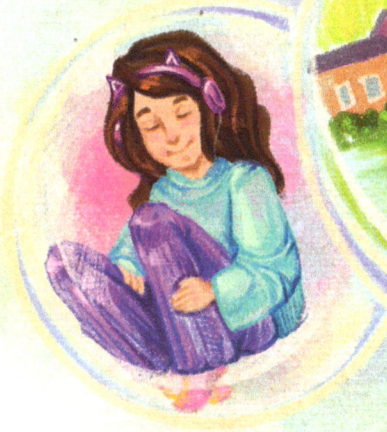

"I can walk to school."

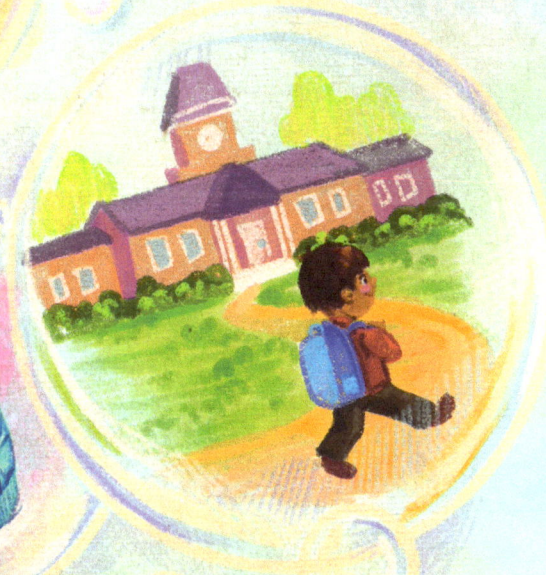

What else can I do?

You are the most powerful part of your care team. Be the superhero you are!

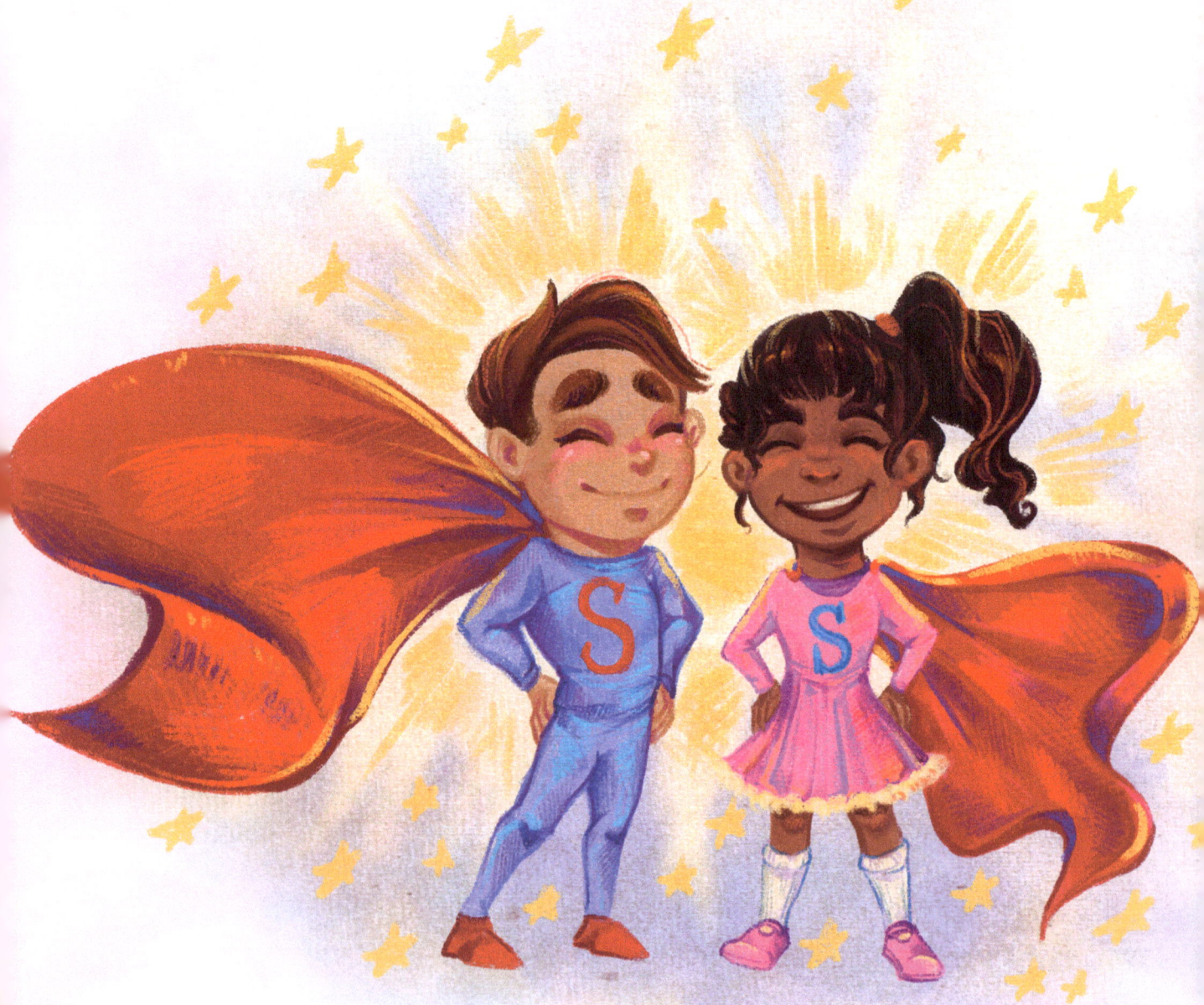

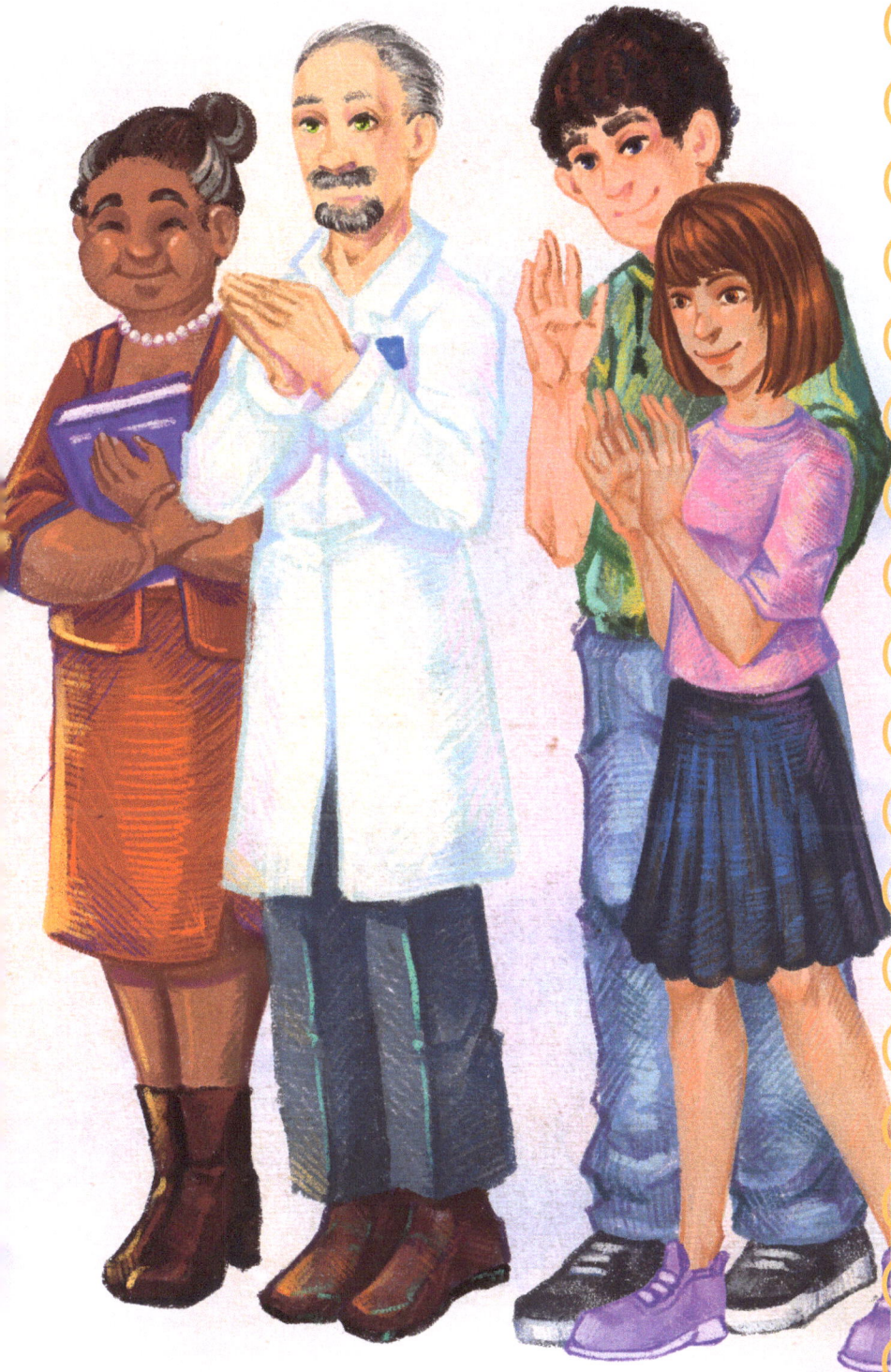

Remember:

Your body and mind need some help to deal with PANS/PANDAS.

You may feel yucky, have new worries, or need to get through procedures you would rather not do.

Everyone is trying to be kind and gentle. You need to be kind and gentle with yourself too.

You need to tell your parents and caregivers:

- **how you feel,**
- **whether you feel better or worse, and**
- **what you need.**

It may change day to day, moment to moment.

Affirmation: *I use my words and try my best to be calm, encourage, and care for myself.*

Remember: Our best is all any of us can do. Sometimes we do better, and sometimes we do worse.

If you have a meltdown, regroup and recover.

Who else helps?

If you suddenly develop new behaviors, or new feelings that are out of control, you need help.

A *psychiatrist* might prescribe medication. Tics, anxiety, out of control anger, depression, and odd movements are caused by the brain being mixed up about its job.

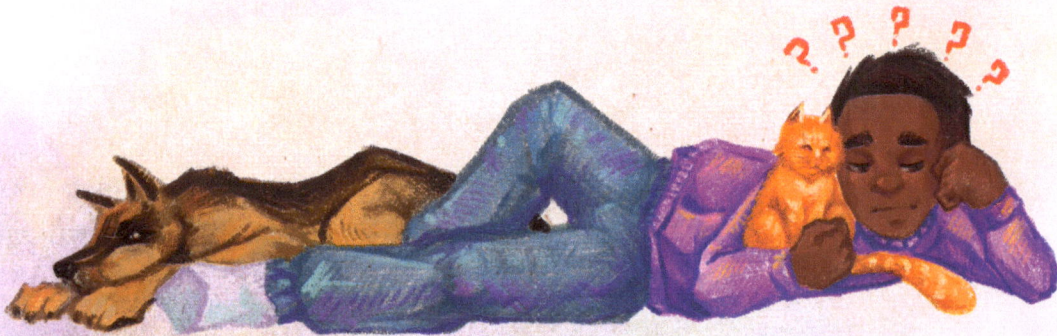

Parents can help

PANS/PANDAS symptoms can be mild, moderate (distressing, impairing but not over the top), or severe (dangerous, life threatening).

Optimistic kids see challenges and obstacles as temporary and able to be overcome.

A chronic illness challenges this.

Remember: they take your words "in," and these words become their inner voice.

Pay attention to all the messages you give, AND all the conversations they hear.

Acknowledge their feelings. Add comfort.

Avoid negativity, or defeatist talk.

Add validation to your child, EVEN as you describe their struggles. Some examples:

- "Tommy's tic is worse in the morning. He tries really hard to get himself up and dressed, even when that is happening."

- "Ava has been washing her hands many times a day. She is doing a great job telling me how it feels when she repeats certain behaviors."

- "You feel _____ (frustrated, scared, upset). How can you get through this (bloodwork, feeling crappy)? How can I help?"

- "What can you be grateful for right now? How can you encourage yourself?"

- "I know we can get through this. Let's make it the best day we can, given how you are feeling?"

You are the example for what you want your child to learn in life. Come up with an action plan.

Remember, children who cope, problem solve, and keep trying until they get through a tough situation become stronger and more capable. Dealing with PANS/PANDAS is a tough situation.

A *psychologist* helps you with feelings, coping skills, learning to tolerate anxiety (decrease obsessiveness), and with communication. They might say, "we are using cognitive behavior therapy." Or, they might do play therapy and they will listen.

The goal is for you and your family to feel more in control, and to have strategies for the challenging times.

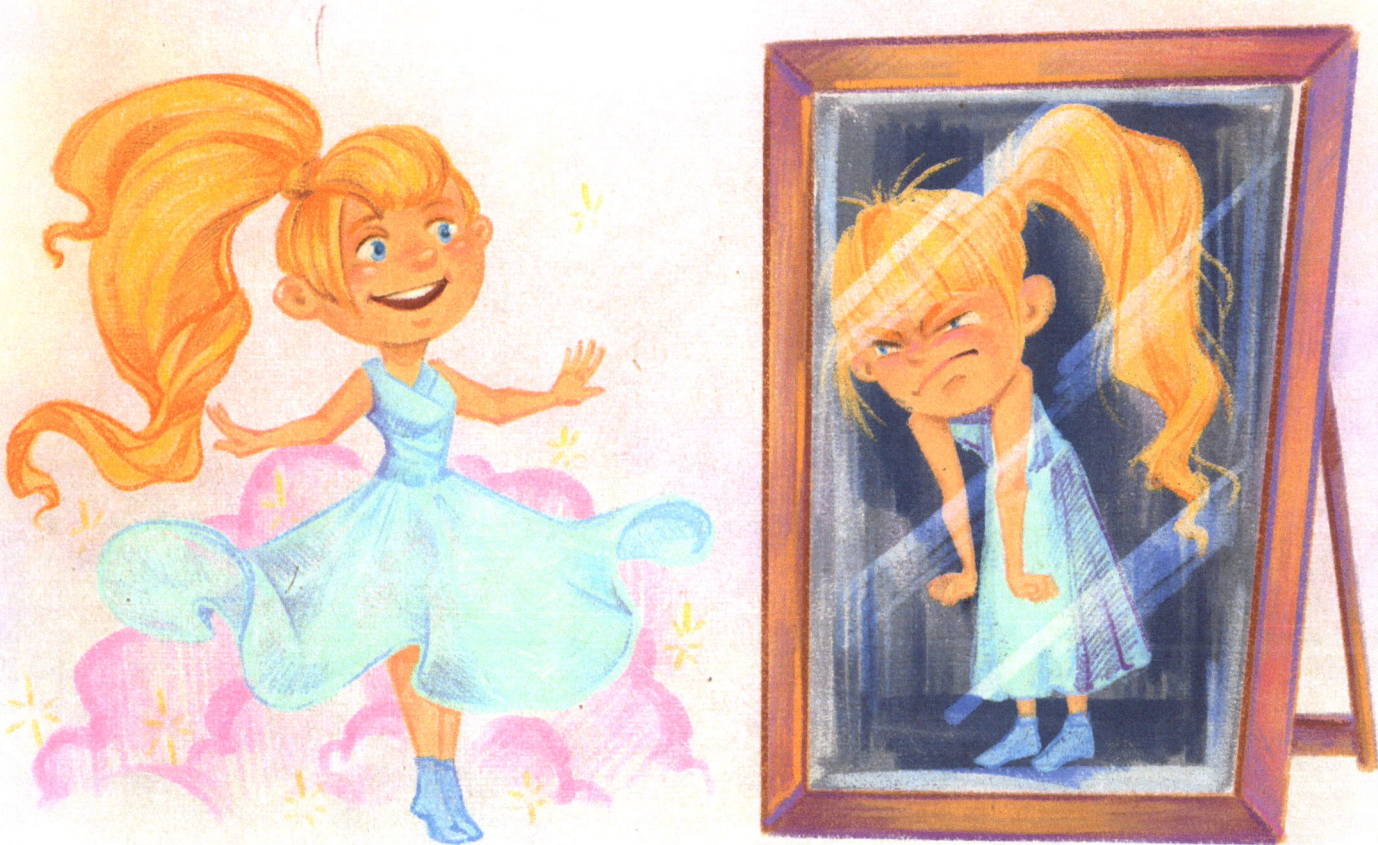

You may feel very different or have new physical and/or emotional challenges.

Being optimistic does not mean you don't have problems. It means you keep looking for the positive in every situation.

Find *anything* positive! For example,

"I did a great job holding still for the x-ray."

"I made it though half a day at school even though I felt yucky. I am awesome."

If you are struggling to do this, ask for help until you learn to do it by yourself.

How can I help my care team help me?

Communicate with your team!

The people in your team need to explain things in language you understand. If they don't, you get to ask them to say it differently.

You also need to give feedback – tell your doctor what is working and what is not.

- **Lately, do you feel better on more days? Worse?**

- **Do you feel better after an infusion?**

- **Are you super grumpy, angry, anxious or depressed?**

- **What would help you right now?**

The whole team's goal is for you to be healthy and happy.

They look busy and rushed sometimes, but you are a priority.

Parents can help

Your child is learning to advocate for themselves. This skill will transfer to other situations in their life.

Make room in doctor visits or during treatments for their voice to be heard. Remember: they do not always get a choice, but a conversation or explanation is helpful to their developing sense of autonomy.

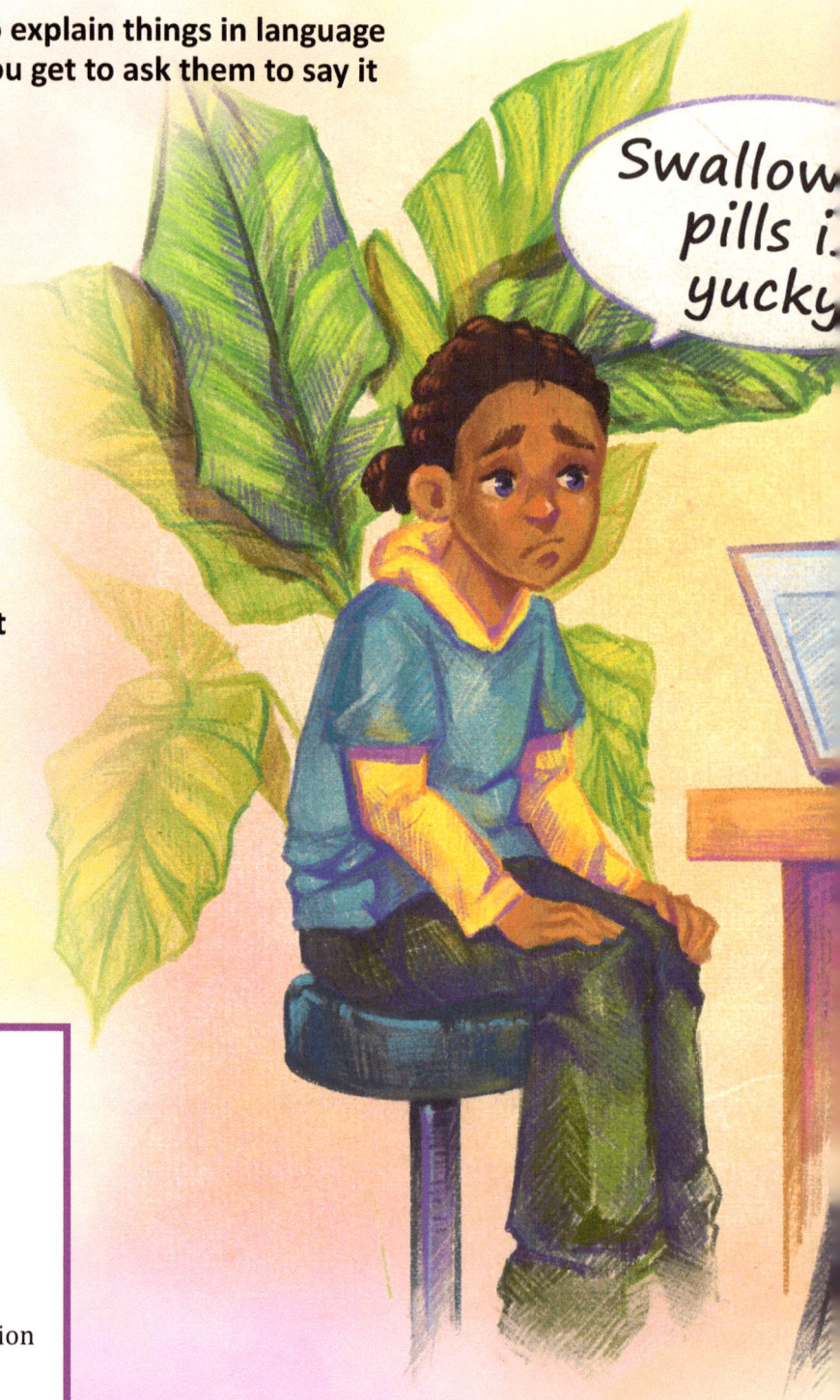

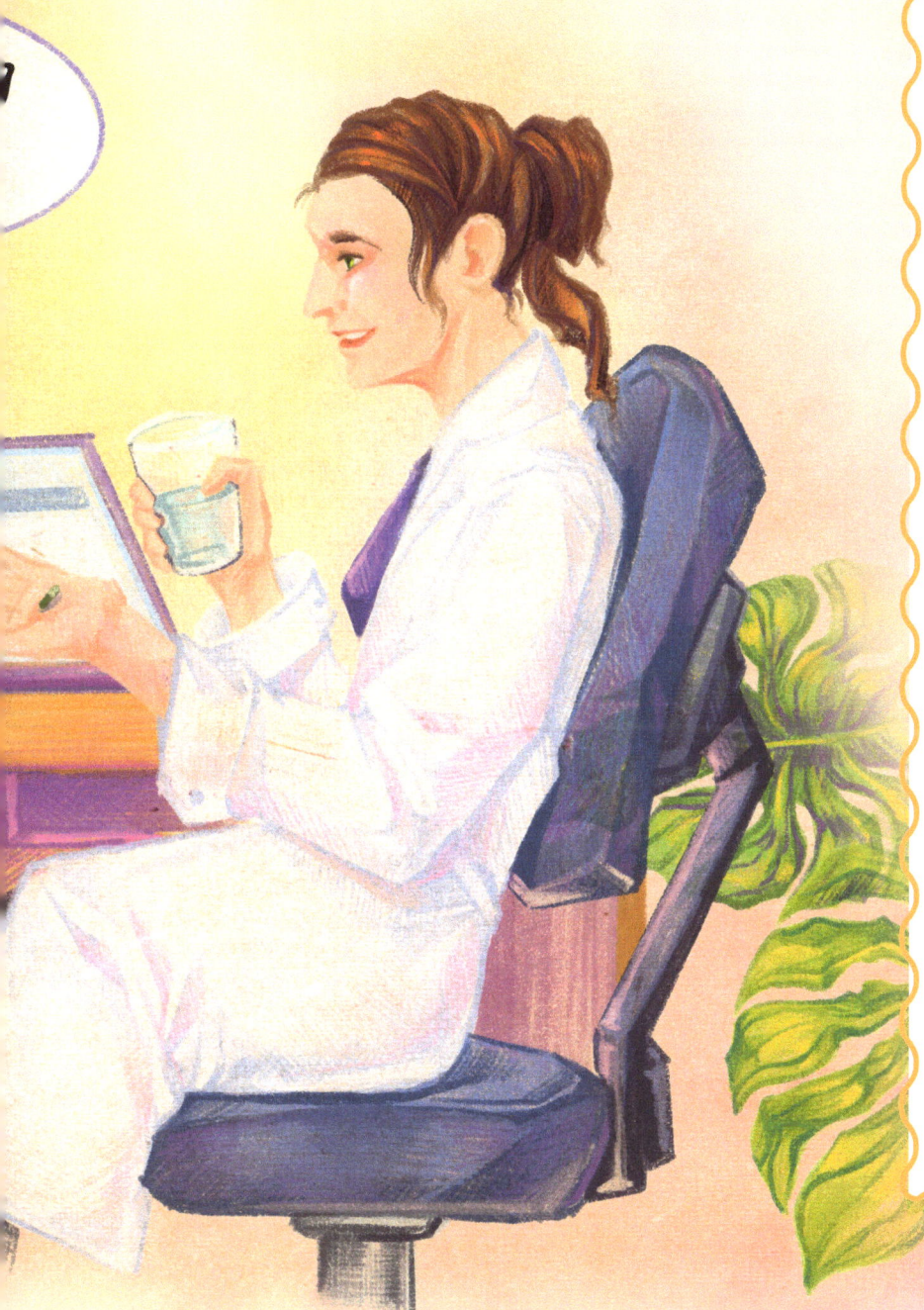

Things for you to say and do:

Listen to your care team. They are cheering for you.

Follow your treatment plan, even if it is yucky sometimes. You are allowed to say,

- "I don't like this," or

- "Swallowing pills is yucky," or

- "Crushed up pills still taste awful," or

- "I will close my eyes during this needle."

You need to express your thoughts and feelings. In fact, that is your job.

All feelings are real feelings, even when they are really BIG feelings.

It is okay to cry. It is okay to be mad.

It is not okay to yell at people.

What about my parents?

When a child develops PANS/PANDAS, it is difficult for everyone to adjust. Your parents know you will have good days and bad days, and it may last a long time. They might get a little grumpy or sad!

Your parents love you. They need strategies, too.

Parents need help, too!

As parents or caregivers, you need a team of trustworthy people to help the family. Your child is strongly affected by how you are managing, by what you do and how you feel. Yes, they sense it. You need to get help, for yourself, for **them.**

You need to start building support for you, your child, and other siblings, **before** you are exhausted, burned out, and overwhelmed.

Everyone needs time to regroup, and rejuvenate, but the caregiver of a sick child needs extra support.

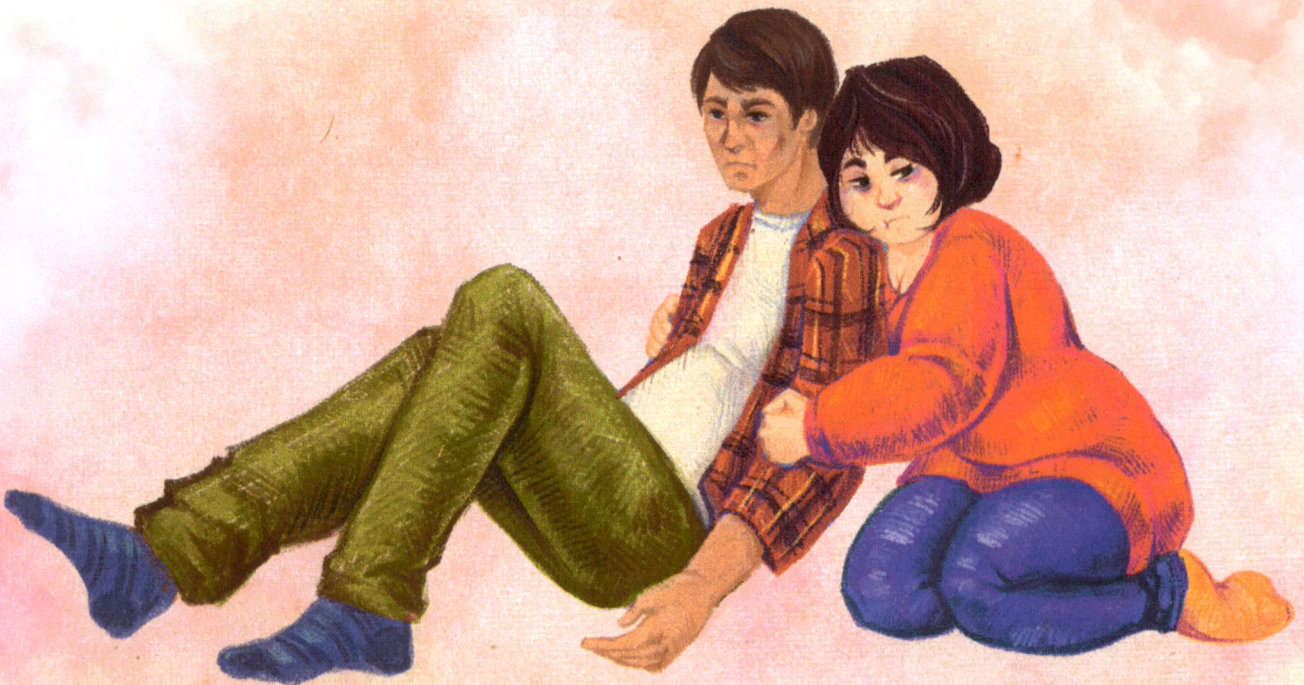

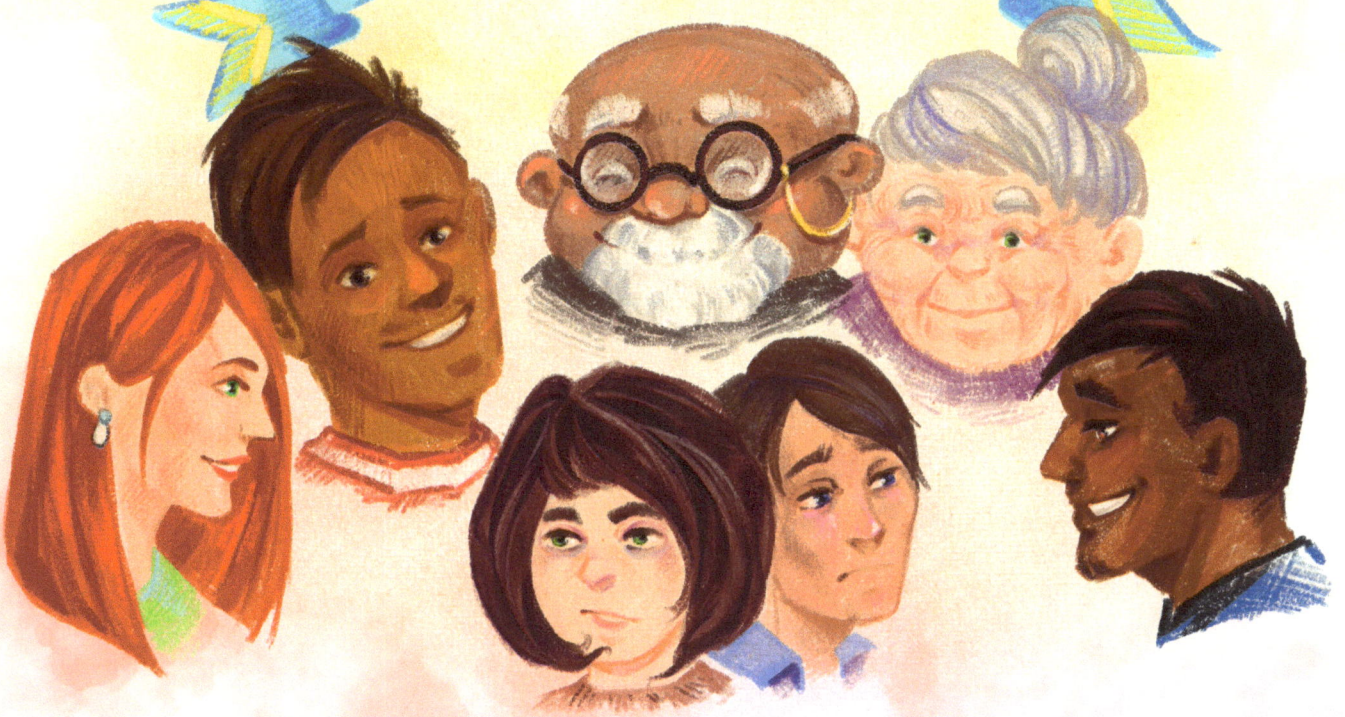

We can help!

How to get support

1. Make a list of potential helpers: moms, dads, grandmas and grandpas, aunts and uncles, friends, neighbors, book club buddies, hockey teammates, parents of children on your kiddo's sports team…

2. Make a schedule.

3. Book people in to spend time with your child or children. Tell them:

   _____ is sick. It is cyclical, and there will be good and bad times.

   We are learning how to handle the illness as a family.

It is not contagious.

I am wondering if you could please …

   … take the kids to school this week (or pick them up)?

   … spend one-to-one time with _____ on Wednesdays from 2 to 5?

   … let me work from home this month, in case ____ needs extra time out of school?

   … make us one casserole every two weeks to help my stress level?

When you ask for help be clear, concise, and specific. Help your support team help you!

Books by Dr. Brayman

Marshmallow the Magic Cat Series

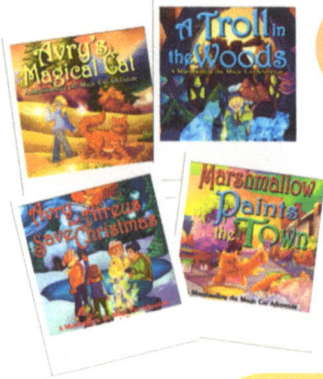

It helps a child to know other kids have troubles, too. This normalizes their struggles and builds empathy. Dr. Brayman's *Marshmallow the Magic Cat* series is about a ten-year-old girl named Avry with anxiety and hypersensitivity. She has many adventures with her magical cat Marshmallow!

8 books available in paperback, e-book and audiobook formats

The Marshmallow series is filled with adventures and real-life themes including collaboration, problem-solving, friendship, dealing with feelings, adventure, overcoming adversity, courage, siblings, introversion, family and more. Each book includes discussion questions at the back.

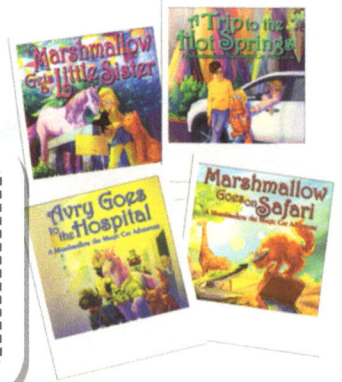

Sibley stories for sleep issues

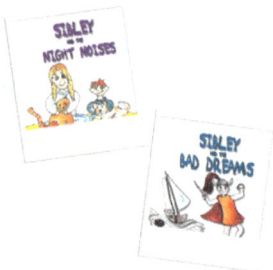

Incorporating all the wisdom of a psychologist and the vivid imagination of a writer, these beautifully illustrated stories help children navigate night time noises and bad dreams.

Loving All of Me for tween and teen girls

Loving All of Me is a therapeutic book, journal and workbook for tween and teen girls, designed to help young women learn how to practice self-love and have a healthy and positive outlook on life and its challenges.

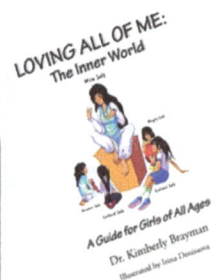

About Dr. Brayman

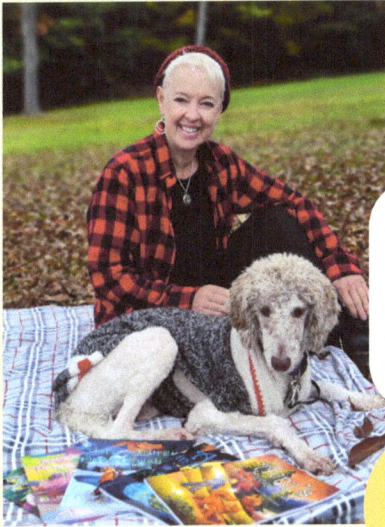

Registered Psychologist

Dr. Kimberly Brayman is a licensed psychologist who resides in Canada. After decades of working in health care, she is inspired to build confidence, normalize struggle, encourage hope, and delight adults and children alike through her storytelling.

Author, Artist, Mother, and Grandmother

She believes stories build empathy and empower the listener to find their own self-reliance and strength. The power of supportive relationships is a strong theme. When a child knows deep in their heart they are loved and accepted, just the way they are, they have a chance to blossom and thrive.

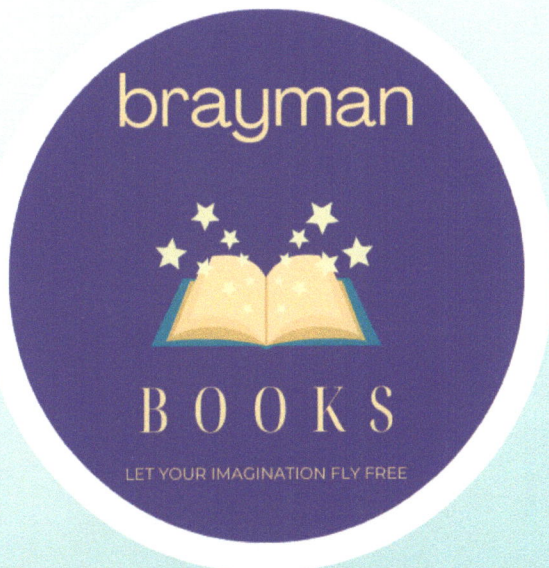

brayman

BOOKS

LET YOUR IMAGINATION FLY FREE

SHOP

BRAYMANBOOKS.COM

FOR ALL OF DR BRAYMAN'S BOOKS

Also available for purchase at

- Amazon
- Kindle
- Audible
- Kobo

see more   @braymanbooks

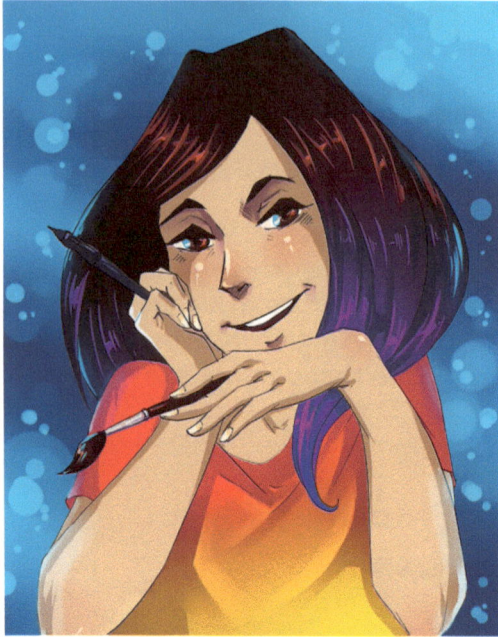

Irina Denissova loves creating illustrations for children's books. Her creative talents bring a magical atmosphere to stories, making them enjoyable for both parents and children. She believes the best part about being an illustrator is that she helps create a new world for readers.

She lives in Temirtau, Kazakhstan and, in her spare time, loves to read and create whatever drawings pop into her mind.

The author describes her as a humble, unbelievably talented young woman who has a near-magical ability to take descriptions and characters and create what the author sees in her own mind.